THE BEST OF NOTES IN ENDOCRINOLOGY: DIABETES SPECIAL

CONTEMPORARY INSIGHTS FROM THE POPULAR BLOG

DR. OM J LAKHANI

Made with ♥ on the Notion Press Platform
www.notionpress.com

"The book is dedicated to the dedicated readers who wholeheartedly supported the first volume"

Contents

Acknowledgements

The inaugural volume of 'Best of Notes in Endocrinology' was met with enthusiasm from readers and endocrinology experts alike. I'm deeply grateful to everyone who supported our work by purchasing the book.

Special thanks to Dr. Sarita Bajaj, who graced us by launching the book at the RSSDI conference in Mumbai in 2023. Her legendary contributions to endocrinology are unparalleled.

This edition, focusing on Diabetes, is inspired by Dr. A. G. Unnikrishnan, CEO and Chief Endocrinologist at Chellaram Diabetes Institute. Known affectionately as 'Dr. Unni sir,' his influence on my life and career is immeasurable. This volume is a tribute to his groundbreaking work in diabetes.

I must also acknowledge Dr. VK Abhichandani's unwavering support. His guidance has been invaluable to my professional journey.

While the previous volume celebrated my family's role, this edition honors my 'Endocrinology family.' Dr. Mohan, Dr. Ameya Joshi, Dr. Basavaraj G S, Dr. Karthik B, Dr. Kaushik Biswas, and Dr. Umesh Garg have been pillars of support and encouragement, greatly contributing to my growth in this field.

Thank you again

Dr. Om J Lakhani

Prologue

Q. What is this book all about?

- *"Notes in Endocrinology"* was an experiment I started to convert my notes into a usable, readable piece of literature for the general public. It is available on Endocrinology.co.in.
- This is t
-
- he first volume featuring some of the best notes from the blog in printed form. It contains nine of the top notes covering various subjects in endocrinology.
- This format caters to those who prefer reading in a traditional manner.

Q. Will "Notes In Endocrinology" continue to exist?

- Yes, the online version will continue.

Q. If these notes are available online, why should I buy this book?

- Good question.
- For two reasons:

1. To support the work we've been doing. The *"Notes in Endocrinology"* is free, but it's a costly project. We need financial support for its continuation. Purchasing this book is a way to support us.
2. Over the years, many have requested a non-digital version of the Notes. So, here it is.

Q. Does this book contain all the notes from the blog?

- No.
- It only features the best of the notes in the field of diabetes
- We also has volume 1 which has a mix bag of notes from Diabetes and Endocrinology

Q. Are these notes a substitute for a textbook?

- No.
- These are supplementary notes. You might still need to refer to textbooks and review articles.

Q. Are these notes a comprehensive review of the given topic?

- They offer a near-complete review of the topic up to the time of publication, but they aren't comprehensive.
- They aren't intended to provide an exhaustive review of the subject.
- Their primary purpose is to serve as notes.

Q. Can you provide a reference for a specific topic?

- Unfortunately, I can't provide references for every point.
- I've included references where possible, but not for every single detail.
- I recognize that this might be an issue for some, but as mentioned, these are notes and not substitutes for actual

research or review articles.

- They might not be perfect; our focus was on simplicity rather than absolute accuracy.
- Remember, these are not peer-reviewed research articles, just notes.

Q. I found an error in the notes. What should I do?

- Errors can occur. If you spot any, please email them to me at dromlakhani@gmail.com, and I'd be grateful for the feedback.

Q. Are more volumes planned for the future?

- The first volume turned out to be economically viable. Hence here is the second volume focussed on diabetes care.
- My goal is to cover the entirety of endocrinology during my lifetime, both on the website and app, and possibly in print.

Q. Do I need to buy volume 1 to read volume 2 ?

- No
- All volumes are independent entities and can be read in any order you like

ONE

PERIOPERATIVE USE OF SGLT2 INHIBITORS

Q. What are the current FDA recommendations for the use of SGLT2i in the perioperative period?

- FDA recommends the following:
    - Stop Canagliflozin, Dapagliflozin, Empagliflozin, and Bexagliflozin at least 3 days before surgery
    - Stop Ertugliflozin at least 4 days before surgery

- Q. What is the basis for the above recommendation in terms of timing?
    - The typical half-life of SGLT2i is 11-13 hours
    - So they are looking at >5 half-lives

- Q. What is the main concern with the use of SGLT2i in the perioperative period?
    - Risk of Euglycemic Ketoacidosis (eDKA)

- Q. What is SAPKA?
    - SGLT2 Inhibitor Associated Perioperative Ketoacidosis (SAPKA)

- Q. When does Euglycemic Ketoacidosis (eDKA) generally occur in these cases?
    - They generally occur in the postoperative period

- Q. True or false, the number of cases reported with Euglycemic Ketoacidosis (eDKA) in literature are increasing over a period of time?
    - True

- Q. What is the definition of Euglycemic Ketoacidosis (eDKA) ?
    - RBS <252 mg/dl with
        - pH <7.3

- Bicarbonate <15 meq/l
- Anion gap >12

- Q. What are the typical Beta-Hydroxybutyrate levels in patients with Euglycemic Ketoacidosis (eDKA) ?
  - Most cases of Euglycemic Ketoacidosis (eDKA) have reported Beta-Hydroxybutyrate levels to be more than 2 mmol/l
  - This is more than 20 mg/dl

- Q. Why do SGLT2i predispose to Diabetic Ketoacidosis ?
  - See the diagram below

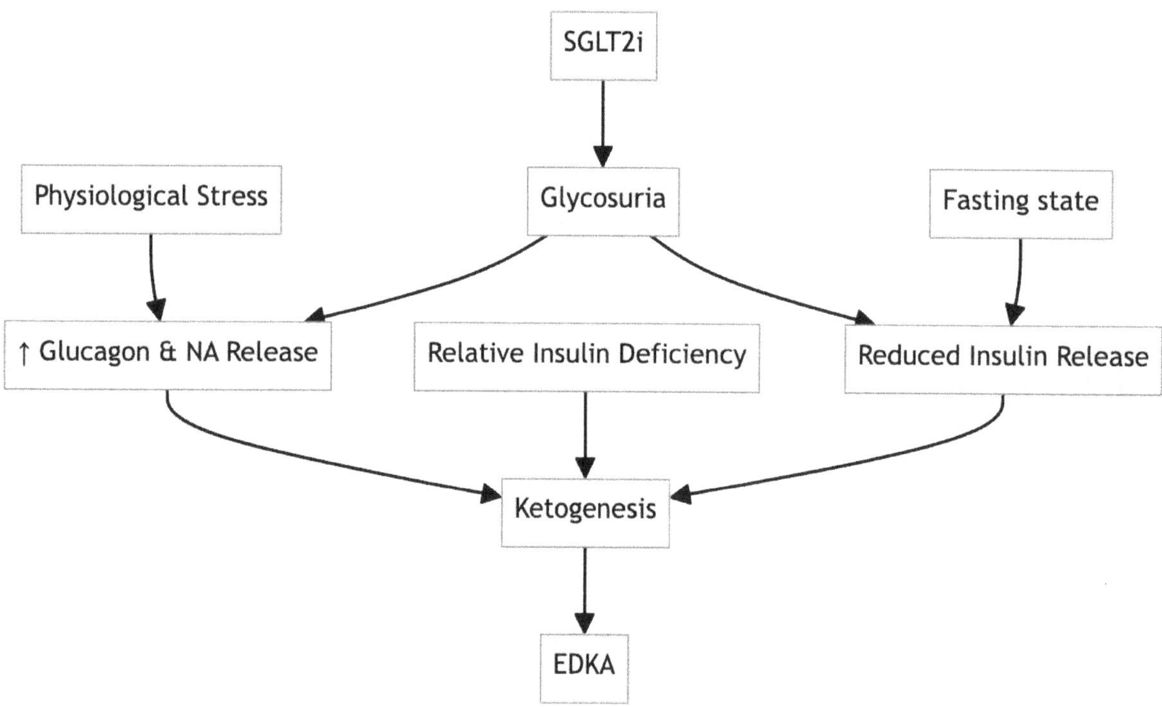

Figure 1.1: Mechanism of Diabetic ketoacidosis due to SGLT2 inhibitors

- Q. Which is the other mechanism recently being recognized as an important cause of increased ketones in patients on SGLT2i?
  - Reabsorption of ketone bodies from urine is seen with the use of SGLT2i
  - This also seems to be an important process in this mechanism

- Q. Do SGLT2i impact Glucagon levels?
  - Yes
  - Patients on SGLT2i have higher glucagon levels
  - However, this impact is indirect

- Q. What are the symptoms of Euglycemic Ketoacidosis (eDKA) ?
  - Symptoms may be more subtle sometimes
    - Respiratory distress
    - Gastrointestinal disturbances
    - Malaise
- Q. What are the key points we have learned about SAPKA from the meta-analysis by Seki et al?
  - Type of Surgery:
    - Bariatric surgery was the most common type of surgery leading to the diagnosis
  - Time to Diagnosis:
    - Most patients (25.3%) were diagnosed on the first postoperative day (POD 1).
  - Trigger for Identification:
    - Laboratory data was the most frequent trigger for identification (29 cases).
    - Nausea and/or vomiting were reported in 21 cases.
    - Breath shortness/dyspnea was a trigger for 20 cases.
    - Fatigue or malaise was reported by 14 patients.
    - Tachycardia and tachypnea were observed in 16 and 15 cases respectively.
  - Blood Ketones and Median BGA Data:
    - The median blood BHB level was 5.8 mmol/L
    - The mean anion gap was 23 meq/l
    - The median pH value at the time of diagnosis was 7.16, with a range from 6.82 to 7.29.
- Q. Do patients receiving SGLT2i for non-diabetes indications like heart failure and CKD are also at risk of Euglycemic Ketoacidosis (eDKA) ?
  - No
  - Non-diabetic patients have NOT been reported to have Euglycemic Ketoacidosis (eDKA)
    - Update- Just one case has been reported as suggested by the meta-analysis by Seki et al (see reference below)
  - Hence in such cases it may be okay to continue SGLT2i preoperatively
  - However they may develop stress hyperglycemia in the perioperative period and hence this has to be kept in mind
  - The guideline recommends getting an anion gap done post-operatively in such patients to rule out Euglycemic Ketoacidosis (eDKA)
- Q. What is the perioperative recommendation for patients with diabetes in whom the SGLT2i have been stopped at an adequate period prior to surgery?

  - The patient can go ahead with surgery with perioperative use of insulin as appropriate
  - However if post-operatively the diet is not resumed within 2 hours it is recommended to get an anion gap done
  - It has to be repeated every 12 hourly after till the carbohydrate in diet is resumed

- Q. Why is this required even for patients in whom the drug has been adequately stopped?
  - This is because the effect of SGLT2i have been shown to persist for a longer time even in patients in whom the drug was discontinued and even with normal renal function
  - Cases of Euglycemic Ketoacidosis (eDKA) have been reported as long as 10 days after discontinuation of the drug

- Q. What to do in diabetic patients on SGLT2i when emergency surgery is required?
  - Check Beta-Hydroxybutyrate and anion gap to ensure that the patient is not currently in DKA
  - If the patient is having DKA- see if emergency surgery can be postponed
  - Else it is recommended to carry out the procedure as usual looking at risk vs benefit

- Q. What is done if the patient shows up for surgery without stopping the medication as suggested?
  - Check anion gap
    - If >12 → postpone surgery
    - If <12 → can go ahead with surgery with good insulinization but make sure that the patient is not having a fasting period of >12 hours

- Q. Give an outline of what to do perioperatively in patients with SGLT2i undergoing surgery?
  - Step 1:

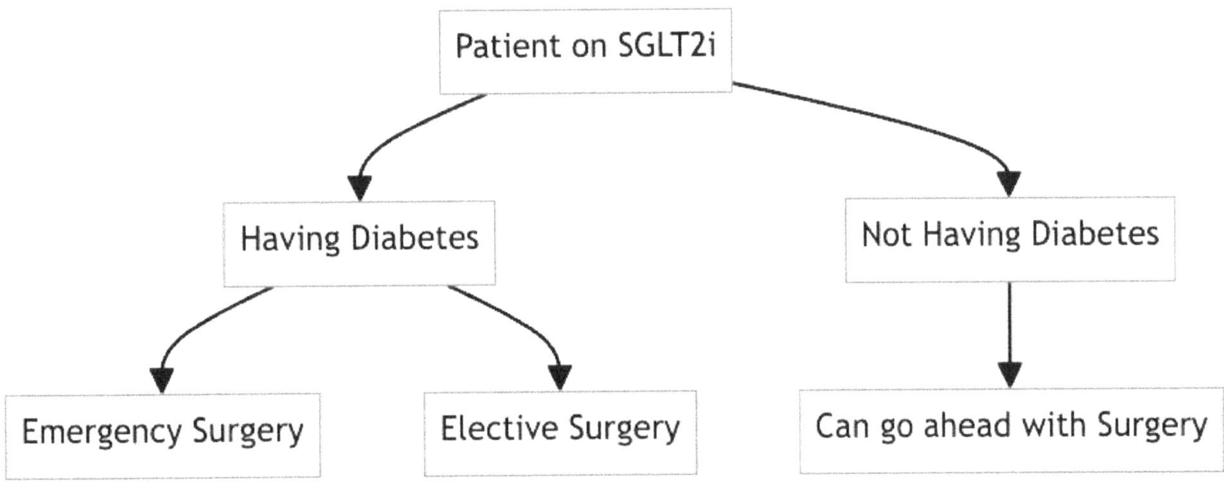

Figure 1.2 : Step 1 in Assessment of Perioperative SGLT2 inhibitor use

- Step 2A - Emergency surgery

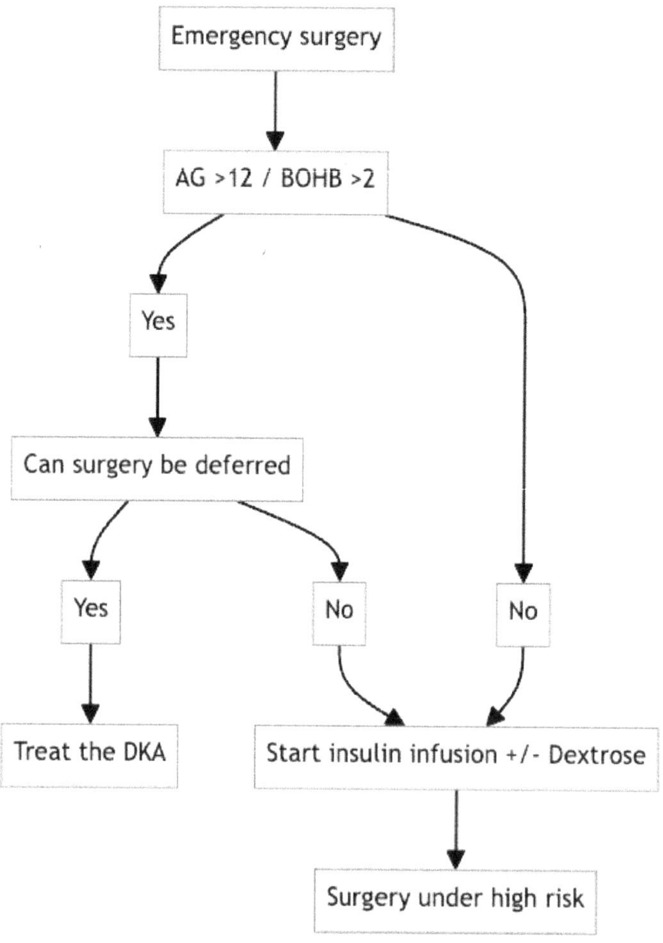

Figure 1.2: Steps taken in Emergency surgery

- Step 2B- Elective surgery

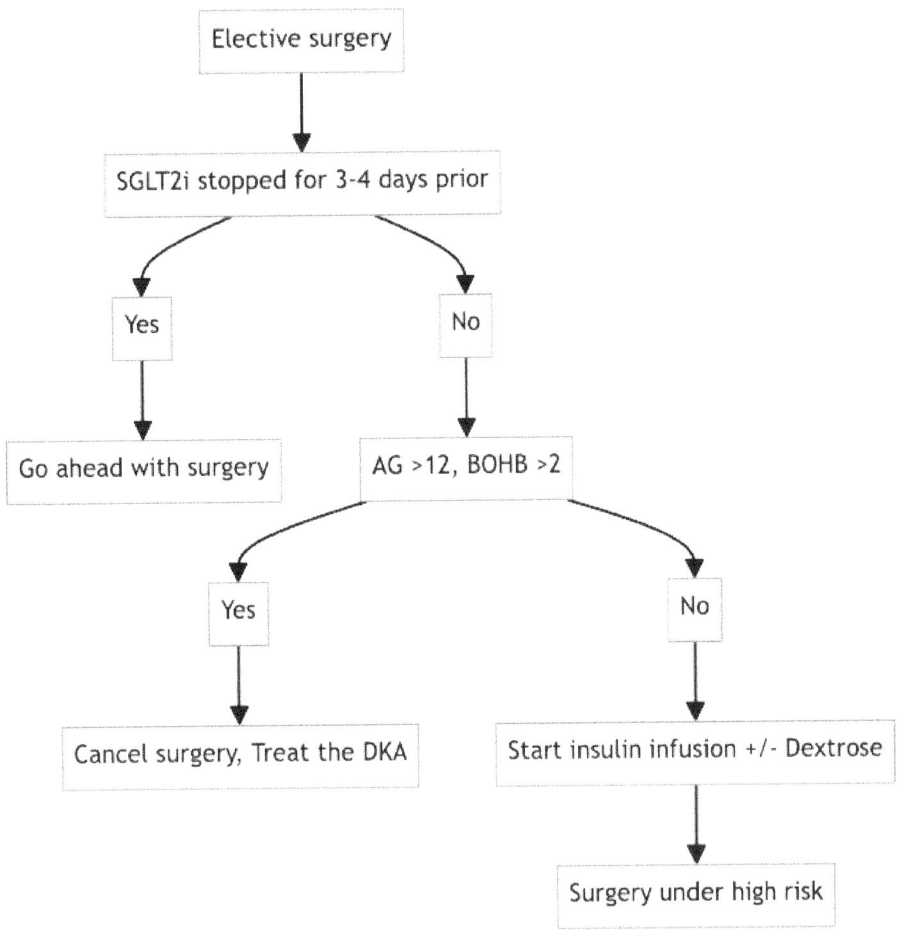

Figure 1.3: Steps taken in Elective surgery

- Q. What should be done intraoperatively in all these patients?
    - Monitor blood glucose and give insulin infusion
        - With dextrose if glucose <200 mg/dl
- Q. What is done post-operatively?
    - It would be a good idea to check the anion gap - if there is going to be a delay of >2 hrs on starting carbohydrate meal
    - If the patient is to be discharged immediately- then it is a good idea to check the glucose and anion gap at discharge- consider insulin if required
        - After the day of the surgery if the patient is taking it orally- they can restart the SGLT2i
    - If the patient is going to be admitted- then continue insulin infusion with dextrose till oral intake is resumed and then put the patient on subcutaneous insulin as per protocol

        - Check the anion gap 4-12 hourly depending on the perioperative risk

- Q. Which surgeries are considered high risk vs low risk in terms of risk of Euglycemic Ketoacidosis (eDKA) ?
    - Factors suggesting low risk:
        - Procedure <1 hr for GA, local or regional anesthesia
        - Total anticipated NPO duration <12 h
        - Pre-op A1C <8%
        - Pre-op blood glucose <150 mg/dl
        - Not on insulin as an outpatient
        - No significant background comorbidity
    - Factors suggesting higher risk:
        - Procedure >1 hour or requiring general anesthesia
        - Total anticipated NPO duration >12 h
        - Pre-op A1C >8
        - Pre-op blood glucose >150 mg/dl
        - On insulin as an outpatient
        - Significant background comorbidity (e.g., trauma, MI, etc).
- Q. How do you manage Euglycemic Ketoacidosis (eDKA) ?
    - Management is the same as other causes of DKA, only that you might have to give dextrose-containing IV fluids since the glucose <250 mg/dl
    - Here is the outline of stepwise management:
        - Step 1: Stop inciting agent, if applicable (e.g., SGLT2i)
        - Step 2: Start fluid replacement with monitoring of electrolytes and ketones
        - Step 3: Start continuous insulin infusion
        - Step 4: Start dextrose administration
- Q. Apart from insulin and dextrose, which drug has been proposed for a potential treatment for Euglycemic Ketoacidosis (eDKA) ?
    - Somatostatin
    - Somatostatin was suggested for the treatment of Diabetic Ketoacidosis way back in 1980 but hasn't been used much because of better insulin available
    - With the advent of Euglycemic Ketoacidosis (eDKA) , the use of the same is emerging as evidenced by the case report by Torre et al
    - The mechanism of action proposed is the reduction of glucagon levels by the use of this agent
- Q. Is there any role of somatostatin analog octreotide in Euglycemic Ketoacidosis (DKA) ?
    - There is mixed data to support the use of Octreotide for this purpose
    - Several papers (Burge et al, Yun et al) have shown little or no benefit of the use of Octreotide in conventional Diabetic Ketoacidosis

- One paper by Diem et al shows that it is useful in preventing recurrence of DKA in patients with recent DKA

ϸϸϸ

References:

1. Raiten JM, Morlok A, D'Ambrosia S, Ruggero MA, Flood J. Perioperative Management of Patients Receiving Sodium Glucose Co-Transporter-2 Inhibitors: Development of a Clinical Guideline at a Large Academic Medical Center. Journal of Cardiothoracic and Vascular Anesthesia. 2023 Oct 10.
2. Torre A, Bisogno N, Botta C, Caiazza A, D'Angelo F, Del Giudice L, Fiorentini P, Marzano L, Nigro R, Sassone D, Torre P. Treatment of a Severe Form of Euglycemic Ketoacidosis in a Patient Treated with SGLT-2 Inhibitors with the Aid of Somatostatin.
3. Burge MR, Qualls CR, Kramer K, Colleran K, Schade DS. Utility of Subcutaneous Octreotide in the Early Recovery from Diabetic Ketoacidosis in Acutely Ill Type 1 Diabetes Patients. J Diabetes Metab Disord Control. 2016;3(5):00079.
4. Yun YS, Lee HC, Park CS, Chang KH, Cho CH, Song YD, Lim SK, Kim KR, Huh KB. Effects of Long-Acting Somatostatin Analogue (Sandostatin) on Manifest Diabetic Ketoacidosis. Journal of Diabetes and its Complications. 1999 Sep 1;13(5-6):288-92.
5. Diem P, Robertson RP. Preventive Effects of Octreotide (SMS 201-995) on Diabetic Ketogenesis during Insulin Withdrawal. Br J Clin Pharmacol. 1991 Nov;32(5):563-7. doi: 10.1111/j.1365-2125.1991.tb03952.x. PMID: 1954071; PMCID: PMC1368631.
6. Ng KE. Management of Euglycemic Diabetic Ketoacidosis.
7. Seki H, Ideno S, Shiga T, Watanabe H, Ono M, Motoyasu A, Noguchi H, Kondo K, Yoshikawa T, Hoshijima H, Hyuga S. Sodium-Glucose Cotransporter 2 Inhibitor-Associated Perioperative Ketoacidosis: A Systematic Review of Case Reports. Journal of Anesthesia. 2023 Feb 27:1-9.

TWO

FROZEN SHOULDER (ADHESIVE CAPSULITIS) IN PATIENTS WITH DIABETES MELLITUS

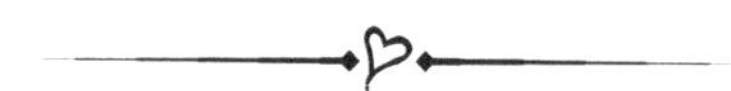

- Q. What is the definition of Frozen shoulder (adhesive capsulitis) ?
  - Frozen shoulder, also known as adhesive capsulitis, is a condition characterized by the gradual development of global limitation of active and passive shoulder motion.
  - It is accompanied by severe shoulder pain.
  - Radiographic findings other than osteopenia are absent in frozen shoulder.
  - It is also referred to as painful stiff shoulder and periarthritis.
- Q. Give me the epidemiology of Frozen shoulder (adhesive capsulitis)
  - It is generally seen in the fifth and sixth decade
  - it is rare before the age of 40 years
  - It is 3 times common in diabetes
  - Women are more affected then men
  - It is generally unilateral
  - It is generally self limiting
  - It is more common in non-dominant arm
- Q. What is the relationship between Frozen shoulder (adhesive capsulitis) and diabetes ?
  - Patients with diabetes mellitus are at a greater risk of developing frozen shoulder.
  - Diabetics are over three times more likely to develop adhesive capsulitis compared to non-diabetics.
  - The overall prevalence of frozen shoulder among diabetics is reported to be 10 to 20 percent.
  - Prevalence of frozen shoulder in patients with long-lasting type 1 diabetes can be as high as 59 percent.
- Q. Does the level of HbA1c predict the likelihood of frozen shoulder ?
  - No
  - According the Yian et at "There was no association found between HbA1c level and the prevalence of frozen shoulder in this diabetic population." (See reference below)

- Q. Which are the other conditions associated with Frozen shoulder (adhesive capsulitis) ?
    - Frozen shoulder has also been associated with thyroid disease, dyslipidemia, prolonged immobilization, stroke, autoimmune disease, Parkinson's disease, and antiretroviral therapy for HIV infection
- Q. What is the pathophysiology of Frozen shoulder (adhesive capsulitis) ?
    - Frozen shoulder, also known as adhesive capsulitis, is characterized by the thickening and tightening of the capsule surrounding the shoulder joint.
    - The exact cause of frozen shoulder is not fully understood, but it is believed to involve a combination of factors including inflammation, fibrosis (formation of excessive scar tissue), and contracture (shortening and tightening) of the joint capsule.
    - Inflammation within the joint leads to the release of inflammatory chemicals, which can cause pain and swelling.
    - Over time, the inflammation triggers the production of excessive scar tissue within the joint capsule, leading to thickening and tightening of the capsule.
    - The thickened and tight capsule restricts the normal movement of the shoulder joint, resulting in pain and stiffness.

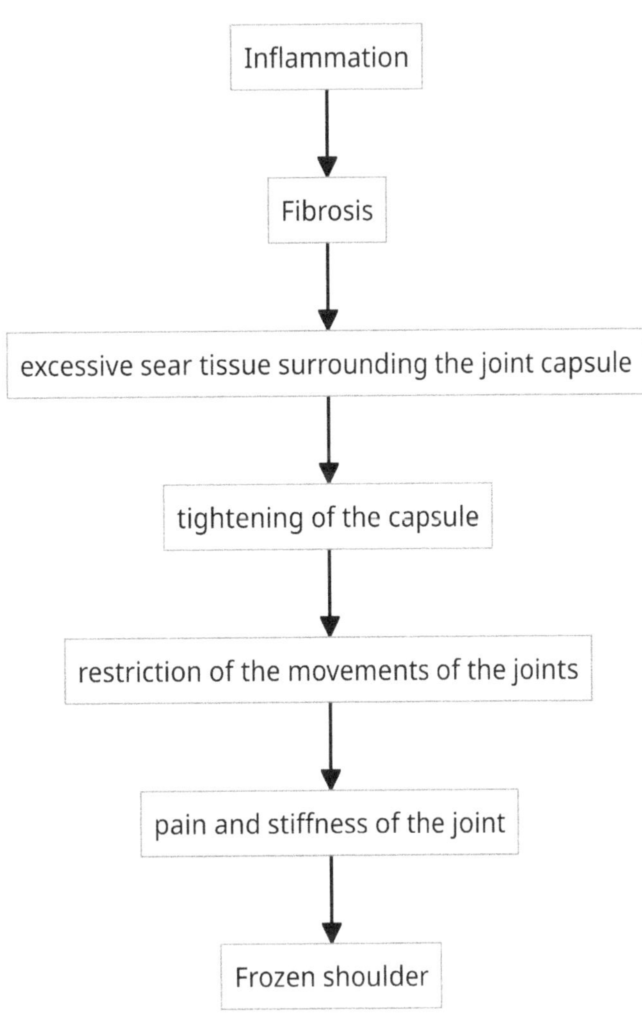

Figure 2.1: Pathophysiology of Frozen shoulder in Diabetes

- Q. Is it similar to Dupuytren's contracture in it's pathophysiology ?
  - It is possible
  - it is also thought that fibrosis is more common in diabetes
- Q. What are the phases of frozen shoulder clinical features ?
  - The phases of frozen shoulder clinical features are as follows:
    - Initial Phase: This phase is characterized by severe and disabling shoulder pain that is worse at night. There is also an increasing stiffness that lasts for two to nine months.
    - Intermediate Phase: In this phase, the pain becomes gradually less pronounced, but there is severe loss of shoulder motion and stiffness. This phase lasts for 4 to 12 months.
    - Recovery Phase: The final phase is marked by a gradual return of range of motion in the shoulder. It takes from 5 to 24 months to complete the recovery phase.
- Q. What are the characteristics of the pain initially felt in patients having frozen shoulder ?
  - So initially there is pain → then loss of motion
  - The pain is typically worse at night
- Q. Which movements of the shoulder joint are typically affected ?
  - External rotation
  - Abduction
  - The patient cannot place the hand on their back or buttock
- Q. Is the restriction of motion due to pain or is it true restriction of motion ?
  - It is true restriction and not just because of pain
- Q. What is the "injection test" ?
  - The injection test is a diagnostic procedure used to distinguish between frozen shoulder and subacromial conditions.
  - It involves injecting an anesthetic into the subacromial space (but outside the joint) to assess the response.
  - In patients with frozen shoulder, active movement restriction and painful end detected with passive motion testing persist after the injection.
  - In contrast, patients with subacromial pathology generally experience pain relief and improved range of motion after the injection.
  - The injection can be performed with or without ultrasound guidance.
- Q. Are investigations necessary for making a diagnosis of Frozen shoulder (adhesive capsulitis) ?
  - No

- Investigations are optional and mainly done to rule out other conditions

- Q. What is the role of performing a plain x-ray in case of a frozen shoulder ?
  - Plain radiographs are generally of limited diagnostic use in patients with frozen shoulder.
  - Most often, the plain film is normal, except for potentially ruling out other disorders such as glenohumeral osteoarthritis.
  - X-rays are not typically necessary to diagnose frozen shoulder.
  - MRI and ultrasound may be more helpful in revealing characteristic changes in the soft tissues consistent with frozen shoulder and assessing the rotator cuff.

- Q. What are the MRI findings in case of frozen shoulder ?
  - MRI has good sensitivity and specificity in making the diagnosis. The findings include
    - Thickening of the coracohumeral ligament and the soft-tissue structures in the rotator cuff interval
    - Coracohumeral ligament thickening
    - Fat obliteration of the rotator cuff interval
    - Enhancement of rotator cuff interval
    - Enhancement of axillary joint capsule
    - Hyperintensity of inferior glenohumeral ligament

- Q. What are the findings on an ultrasound ?
  - Thickening of the coracohumeral ligament and the soft-tissue structures in the rotator cuff interval (in the early phase)

- Q. How will you differentiate clinically frozen shoulder from subacromial conditions ?
  - Patients with subacromial conditions often have a history of heavy lifting or repetitive movements, especially above shoulder level.
  - Patients with subacromial conditions often complain of activity-related pain and problems performing usual activities.
  - Limitations in shoulder motion are more often due to pain in patients with subacromial conditions, as opposed to the mechanical restrictions found with frozen shoulder.
  - Patients with frozen shoulder may have a spontaneous onset without an apparent cause or a history of overuse or abnormal activity.
  - Frozen shoulder can develop following shoulder injuries, surgery, or prolonged immobilization for any reason.
  - Patients with frozen shoulder often complain of chronic, severe, nagging pain deep in the shoulder joint, especially at night.
  - Age can be a distinguishing factor, as frozen shoulder is unlikely in patients younger than 40 years of age, while patients older than 70 are more likely to have rotator cuff tears or glenohumeral osteoarthritis

- Q. What is the important difference between these conditions in terms of range of motion ?
  - In subacromial condition, the limitation of motion is mainly due to pain
  - Hence there is reduction in active range of motion but passive range of motion is preserved

- However in case of frozen shoulder - the restriction is due to pain as well as actual restriction in movement and hence both active and passive range of motion is affected
- Physiotherapy is helpful after the initial painful phase is over

- Q. What is the principal of management of Frozen shoulder (adhesive capsulitis) ?

    - It is generally self resolving and does not need any treatment in most cases

- Q. What treatment can be offered for moderate to severe pain ?]

    i. Intra-articular glucocorticoids
    ii. Suprascapular nerve block

- Q. What is role of physiotherapy in Frozen shoulder (adhesive capsulitis) ?

    - Physical therapy is commonly used to treat frozen shoulder.
    - Evidence for the effectiveness of physical therapy is limited.
    - A meta-analysis of 32 trials found that the efficacy of manual therapy or exercise remains unclear, with most studies reporting no significant differences among treatment groups.
    - One study suggested that exercise performed within the limits of pain led to greater improvements in shoulder function than intensive physical therapy.
    - More aggressive stretching of the shoulder muscles and capsule may be useful in the later phase of the condition.
    - The addition of supervised physical therapy following an intraarticular injection of glucocorticoid may result in more rapid improvement than injection alone.
    - Patients with mild disease and those early in the recovery phase of frozen shoulder may benefit from performing gentle range of motion exercises, such as pendulum swings, as long as they do not cause undue discomfort.
    - To summarize- physical therapy is useful- but only more gentle exercises rather than more aggressive situations

- Q. What kind of shoulder motion exercises are recommended ?

    - Gentle abduction
    - Gentle external rotation
    - Gentle internal rotation
    - Abduction-adduction with exercise band
    - Flexion-extension with exercise band
    - Seated external rotation with elbow resting on table

- Q. What is the role of oral glucocorticoid therapy ?

    - Oral glucocorticoid therapy is not recommended as a routine treatment for frozen shoulder.
    - Intraarticular glucocorticoid injections are more effective than oral glucocorticoids for treating frozen shoulder.
    - Oral glucocorticoids may have potential adverse effects.
    - Intraarticular glucocorticoid injections lead to improved range of motion and pain relief in frozen shoulder.

- Q. What is the role of intraarticular glucocorticoid injection ?
    - Intraarticular glucocorticoid injections are beneficial in the treatment of frozen shoulder.
    - They can lead to improved range of motion and pain relief. However, the benefits are temporary
    - Multiple injections may be beneficial, with up to three injections showing evidence of effectiveness.
    - Adverse reactions may include increased pain after injection, facial flushing, rash, and irregular menstrual bleeding.
    - Sonographic guidance for intraarticular injections is being used more frequently and may improve effectiveness.
    - Further randomized trials are needed to test the hypothesis of ultrasound-guided injections and alternative injection sites.
    - Pending the results of such studies, it is suggested to use intraarticular injections.
- Q. What is the role of glucocorticoid injection combined with physical therapy ?
    - Glucocorticoid injection combined with physical therapy may be more effective than either therapy alone for frozen shoulder.
    - It can result in faster improvements in shoulder function compared to other treatment approaches.
    - The combination therapy has shown to provide pain relief, improve range of motion, and reduce disability.
    - Evidence supporting the effectiveness of glucocorticoid injection combined with physical therapy is limited but promising.
- Q. What is the role of suprascapular nerve block ?
    - Suprascapular nerve block can reduce the pain associated with early frozen shoulder.
    - It may provide additional benefits by addressing the involvement of the suprascapular nerve in the pathophysiology of frozen shoulder.
    - A systematic review and meta-analysis showed significant improvements in pain, motion, and overall shoulder function following a suprascapular nerve block.
    - In a randomized trial, patients treated with a suprascapular nerve block in addition to glenohumeral injection and physical therapy experienced reduced pain, increased mobility, and a resolution of symptoms six months sooner than patients treated with glenohumeral injection and physical therapy alone.
- Q. What is intraarticular dilatation ?
    - Intraarticular dilatation, also known as hydrodilatation or arthrographic distension, is a treatment for frozen shoulder.
    - It involves combining an intraarticular injection of an anesthetic with an infusion of saline to dilate the glenohumeral capsule.
    - Saline is injected into the joint under pressure to increase joint volume and improve glenohumeral motion.
    - It is based on the finding that frozen shoulder involves thickening and contraction of the glenohumeral joint capsule and surrounding collagenous tissue, leading to reduced joint volume.
    - Studies have shown that arthrographic distension with saline and glucocorticoid provides short-term benefits in pain reduction, range of motion, and overall shoulder function in patients with frozen shoulder.
- Q. What is the role of surgery in these cases ?
    - Surgical referral should be deferred as long as the patient is making progress with nonoperative management.

- Surgery should be reserved for patients who do not respond to conservative management.
- There are no formal guidelines to determine the appropriate timeframe for surgical referral.
- Most patients should be managed conservatively for at least 10 to 12 months, as long as they are making progress.

• Q. What type of surgery is done in such cases ?

- Arthroscopic release of adhesive capsulitis
- Manipulation under anesthesia

• Q. In patients with diabetes mellitus and frozen shoulder, how does good glycemic control improve the outcomes ?

- Currently there is no evidence to suggest that improvement in glycemic control leads to improved outcomes in patients with Frozen shoulder (adhesive capsulitis)

❧❧❧

References:

1. Yian EH, Contreras R, Sodl JF. Effects of glycemic control on prevalence of diabetic frozen shoulder. J Bone Joint Surg Am. 2012 May 16;94(10):919-23. doi: 10.2106/JBJS.J.01930. PMID: 22617920.

THREE

Treatment of Diabetic Neuropathy

- Q. What are the three main aspects of management of Diabetic neuropathy ?
    - Glycemic control
    - Foot care
    - Treatment of pain

GLYCEMIC CONTROL

- Q. Does glycemic control IMPROVE diabetic neuropathy?
    - This is an area of debate
    - Many studies including DCCT have shown objective improvement in glycemic control including improvement in VPT and NCV
    - At present, however, it is believed that once established, diabetic neuropathy cannot be reversed and only progression can be halted by good glycemic control
- Q. What type of neuropathy can be corrected with glycemic control alone?
    - Acute painful diabetic neuropathy and rapidly reversible hyperglycemic neuropathy – can be corrected with glycemic control alone
    - However, in some cases, rapid improvement in glycemic control can lead to "insulin neuritis"
    - Hence stable glycemia is the aim not under or overtreatment

FOOT CARE

- Q. What are the components of foot care for diabetics?
    - Daily inspection of feet by patients
    - Physician inspection on regular visits

MANAGEMENT OF PAINFUL DIABETIC NEUROPATHY

- Q. What are the points of difference between neuropathic pain from ischemic pain in diabetics?

	Neuropathic	Ischemic
Location of pain	feet	Calf
Nature of pain	Sharp tingling	Deep ache
walking	Relives pain	Worsens pain
rest	Worsens pain	Relives pain
Nightime	Pain is worse	Pain is better
History of recent change in glycemic status	present	Absent

Table 3.1: Difference between Neuropathic and Ischemic pain

- Q. Does the painful neuropathy spontaneously resolve?
    - In 55% of cases the pain resolves in 12 months
    - This is especially true if there is a recent change in glycemic status and there is a history of painful acute sensory neuropathy which is generally self-resolving
- #Pearl
    - Nerve may discharge spontaneously when it is either being damaged or being repaired
- Q. Does the pain disappear always a good sign?
    - Disappearance of pain can mean either there is improvement in the nerve function or deterioration
    - It is not always a good thing

PAIN CONTROL

- Q. Enlist the drugs used in the management of Painful diabetic neuropathy.
    - Antidepressants

    - Amitriptyline
    - Duloxetine
    - Venlafaxine
    - Desipramine

  - Anticonvulsants

    - Pregabalin
    - Gabapentin
    - Valproate

  - Others

    - Isorbidade dinitrate spray
    - Capsaicin cream
    - Alpha lipoic acid
    - TENS- transcutaneous electric nerve stimulation

- Q. Which are the three first-line agents in painful diabetic neuropathy?

  - SNRI- duloxetine, and venlafaxine
  - TCA- Amitryptiline , nortyptiline and desipramine
  - Gabapentinoid antiseizure medications - pregabalin , gabapentin

- Q. Of the above which is the best medication?

  - No medication is better than other
  - Hence the choice should depend on comorbidities, side effect profile, and patient preferences

- Q. Are antidepressants effective?

  - Yes
  - They have been proven in clinical trials
  - Effect is generally seen in 6 weeks and the dose required is less than the dose typically used in depression

- Q. What are the common side effects of amitriptyline and duloxetine?

  - Amitriptyline – Dry mouth
  - Duloxetine – constipation

- Q. What is the typical dose of amitriptyline used?

  - Starting dose of 10-25 mg
  - Can give up to 100 mg/day
  - Given at bedtime

- Q. In which patients do you need to be careful while prescribing TCA?

  - Patient with a history of heart disease

- Q. Which is the least cardiotoxic TCA?
  - Doxepin
- Q. Which TCA has fewer anticholinergic side effects?
  - Nortriptyline
- #Pearl
  - Also, be careful of using amitryptiline in elderly males – as they can have urinary retention if they have a prostate problem. In patients with prostate issue, Amitryptiline can be replaced by nortriptyline
- Q. What is the action of Duloxetine?
  - It is a combination of SNRI and SSRI
- Q. What is the important side effect of duloxetine in diabetics?
  - It can cause a mild increase in blood glucose
- Q. What is the typical dose of Duloextine used?
  - Typically used in a dose of 60 mg
  - Starting dose of 20-30 mg - escalate up to 120 mg
  - Must be taken on a full stomach
- Q. Why is the drug given on empty stomach?
  - It can cause nausea as an important side effect
- Q. Can it be combined with other SNRI?
  - No
  - But it can be combined with pregabalin
- Q. In which related condition, it must be avoided?
  - Avoid patients having restless leg syndrome since it can exacerbate the problem in such patients
- Q. What is the mechanism of action of Pregabalin?
  - Inhibits presynaptic release of excitatory neurotransmitters
- Q. What is a common but important side effect of Pregabalin?

- Weight gain
- Typically about 7% of weight gain is seen
- Does not impact diabetes control

- Q. How do you dose pregabalin ?
  - Typical starting dose is 75-150 mg/day
  - Generally given in 2-3 divided doses
  - Most trials use a starting dose of 150 mg/day
  - Every 3-7 days, 75 mg dose can be increased to upto 300 mg/day
  - For other indications up to 600 mg/day is given, but for neuropathy 300 mg/day is generally sufficient
- Q. Is it a habit-forming drug?
  - Yes
- Q. Is gabapentin useful in painful diabetic neuropathy?
  - Yes. However, some trials have shown mixed results
  - Trials have shown it is not effective as placebo
  - It is typically given in a dose of 300-600mg TID
- Q. Which other anticonvulsants can be used?
  - Valproate and carbamazepine are effective but generally not used because of better drugs are available
- Q. What is the mechanism of action of Capsascian cream?
  - It causes local depletion of substance P
- Q. How and when is it used?
  - It is available as 0.075% cream
  - It is applied topically 4 times a day
  - Generally used if anticonvulsants and antiepileptics don't work
- Q. What is the logic of using alpha lipoic acid (ALA) in DN?
  - ALA is an antioxidant
  - We know the role of reactive oxygen species in the etiology of DN
- Q. Which are the important trials with ALA?
  - SYDNEY 1 trial- IV ALA
  - SYDNEY 2 trial- use oral ALA
  - These trials have shown ALA to be effective
- Q. What is the dose of oral ALA to be used?

- Oral ALA in a dose of 600 mg OD can be used in cases refractory to other medications

- Q. Which opioids have been used?
    - Tramadol
    - Oxycodone
    - Dextromethorphan
    - However, they are best avoided as they can cause addiction

- Q. Are combination treatments more effective than a single drug?
    - Yes

- Q. Is transcutaneous electric nerve stimulation useful?
    - Yes
    - TENS is useful for diabetic neuropathy

- Q. What about acetyl L carnitine?
    - Some trials have shown it to be effective in a dose of 1000 mg

- Q. Which spray is effective?
    - Isorbidade dinitrate spray
    - Small trials have shown it to be effective

- Q. What is the role of NSAIDs?
    - NSAIDs are effective in reducing pain in diabetic neuropathy
    - However, it can worsen nerve injury hence it is better avoided than other meds

- Q. Which procedure is used in refractory DN?
    - Spinal cord stimulation
    - It is an invasive procedure
    - Electrodes were introduced to give nerve stimulation to a dorsal column of the spinal cord

- Q. Which drug according to the American academy of neurology is most effective?
    - Pregabalin – in dose of 300-600 mg/day

- Q. What is the ADA approach?
    - 1st- Rule out non-diabetic etiology
    - 2nd - Stabilize blood glucose
    - 3rd- Tricyclic antidepressants / anticonvulsants
    - 4th- Opioid and other agents

NON-GLYCEMIC MEASURES

- Q. What is the role of surgical decompression?
  - It is known as Dellon's procedure
  - It is the decompression of peripheral nerves as a treatment of painful diabetic neuropathy
  - However it is controversial and not recommended
- Q. Which anti-diabetic drug used in diabetes produces B12 deficiency?
  - Metformin
- Q. What B12 level is optimal in diabetic patients?
  - Generally -250 pg/ml
  - In diabetics – 460 pg/ml is the optimal B12 level
- Q. Which B12 preparation is better for diabetics?
  - Methylcobalamin Is better for diabetics, not cyanocobalamin
  - It is given in a dose of 3000 ug/day which achieves a B12 level of 1000 pg/ml
- Q. Which 2 conditions are often associated with painful Diabetic neuropathy ?
  - Mood disorder
  - Sleep disorder
  - Hence the treatment should address these issues as well
- Q. Apart from tramadol which is the other centrally acting opioid?
  - Tapentadol
  - It is available in India as TYDOL

FOUR
GLYCATED HEMOGLOBIN (HBA1C)

- Q. Who was the first to describe HbA1c?
    - Rhabar et al
- Q. What is the most appropriate Term for HbA1c?
    - It is glycated hemoglobin and not glycosylated hemoglobin
    - Glycosylated suggests it is an enzymatic process whereas, in reality, it is a non-enzymatic reaction
- Q. What does 1c stand for in HbA1c ?
    - 1c stands for the order of hemoglobin molecules on electrophoresis
- Q. On what chain of the hemoglobin is the glucose added?
    - It is added to the beta-chain of the hemoglobin
- Describe the steps to HBA1c formation.
    - Glucose binds to the N terminal of valine residue on the Beta chain of HbA
    - Formation of Schiff's bases (Aldimine) non-enzymatically →
    - Converts to Amadori product (Irreversible ketamine) →
    - Intermediate glycosylation production →
    - Cross-links- Advanced glycosylation end products
- Q. What part of the above reaction are we measuring when we measure HbA1c?
    - We are measuring the irreversible ketoamine and not the Schiff's base aladmine
    - The Aldimine is transient and reflects acute glucose fluctuation
    - While the Ketoamine is irreversible and represents chronic hyperglycemia
- Q. HbA1c reflects what period of glycemic control?
    - It reflects truly the glycemic control of only the last 8 weeks
    - Even though the idea is that it lasts the entire period of RBC which is 120 days in reality it only lasts for 8 weeks

- 50% of the HbA1c is formed in the last 1 month and that of last 3-4 months only contribute 10%

- Q. What are more glycated – The older RBCs or reticulocytes?
    - The older RBCs are more glycated than reticulocytes

HBA1C ASSAYS AND METHODS

- Q. Describe the various methods for HbA1c estimation.

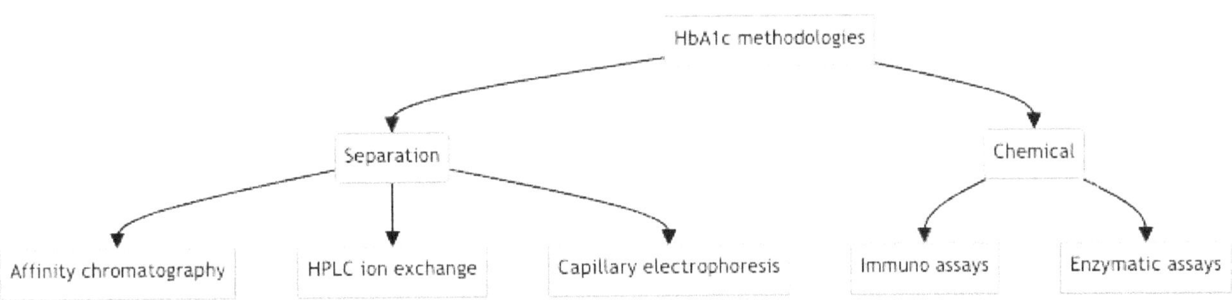

Figure 4.1: Different methods for HBA1c estimation

- Q. Which assay was used in the DCCT trial?
    - It used D10 cation exchange HPLC
    - To be specific- BIORAD DIAMAT using Bio-Rex 70 resin was used in DCCT and also UKPDS

- Q. What is ADAG?

- It is the study that came up with the estimated average glucose (eAG) formula for HbA1c
- The study was called "A1c Derived glucose"

- Q. What is the ADAG formula?
  - eAG = 28.7 x HbA1c – 46.7

STANDARDIZATION

- Q. What is the difference between standardization and harmonization?
  - Harmonization- calibrating the assay using an arbitrarily chosen standard
  - Standardization- calibrating the assay using a standard that is of high order
- Q. What is the current standardization process for HbA1c?
  - Old standardization was done by NGSP (National Glycohemoglobin Standardization Program) which standardized using an assay that was used in DCCT
  - This assay was an HPLC ion exchange electrophoresis
  - It reported as % of total hemoglobin
  - It was harmonization and not standardization
  - The newer standardization is given by IFCC (international federation for clinical chemists)
  - It is a different assay
  - It reports the value as mmol/mol
- Q. How is the IFCC reference derived?
  - 3 steps
  - Step 1
    - Hb separated from lysed RBC is cleaved using endoproteinase
  - Step 2
    - The glycated and non-glycated particles are separated using HPLC
  - Step 3
    - The glycated particles which are separated are measured using capillary electrophoresis
- Q. How is the current reporting done?
  - According to the current consensus the reporting is to be done in three formats
  - IFCC – using mmol/mol value
  - NGSP - % value
  - eAG from ADAG formula

- Q. What is the relation between the new assay of IFCC and DCCT assay?
  - The new assay gives a value that is 1.5% lower than the older assay
- Q. How is the NGSP value of % divided by the IFCC value?
  - Using the formula 0.0914 * IFCC + 2.152
- Q. Using the formula what is HbA1c <7 % in IFCC terms?
  - It is around 53 mmol/mol
- Q. Which anticoagulant is used while taking an HbA1c blood sample?
  - EDTA
- Q. What should the CV be for HbA1c?
  - Interlaboratory - CV <3%
  - Intralaboratory -CV <5%

FALSE VALUES

- Q. What are the common causes of false high and false low values of HbA1c?
  - False High
    - Iron deficiency anemia
    - B12 and folic acid deficiency
    - CKD (uremia)- carbamylated hemoglobin
    - Asprin
    - HbF and HbG
  - False low
    - HbS and HbC
    - Hemolytic anemia
    - Pregnancy
- Q. Do the Hemoglobin variants always create a problem?
  - No
  - The newer HPLC and Capillary electrophoresis methods tend to separate the Hb variants and hence do not interfere with the test results
  - The chemical methods do not normally separate the Hb variants

- Q. What happens in CKD?
    - Carbamylated Hb- false high
    - Increase hemolysis and use of EPO - false low
- Q. What are the racial differences in HbA1c?
    - They are uncertain
    - But Africans and Hispanics- Higher HbA1c
    - Asian and Caucasians- lower HbA1c
- Q. What is the relation between HBA1c and age?
    - With every decade of life HBA1c increase by 0.1% or 1 mmol/mol
- Q. Why does HbA1c correlate so well with Diabetic microvascular complications
    - Glucose enters the RBC via the GLUT1 channel
    - here is bonds to the N-terminus of the Hemoglobin beta-chain to produce an HbA1c
    - Glucose also enters the tissue in which microvascular complications are seen via GLUT1
    - hence the glucose levels intracellular in these organs (kidney, retina, neurons) are similar to that in RBC
    - hence HbA1c correlates well with microvascular complications
- Q. What is the Glycation gap?
    - glycation gap is the difference between the measured HbA1c and the predicted HbA1c
    - this article writes that in almost 30% of patients with Type 1 Diabetes - the HbA1c values do not correlate with the measured SMBG values!
- Q. Does the type of sample- arterial, venous, or capillary affect the results?
    - No data regarding arterial, but generally capillary testing is similar to venous
    - the difference is NOT significant
- Q. Does point-of-care testing for HBA1c give inferior results?
    - Not necessarily
- Q. Does HbA1c show diurnal variation ?
    - No
- Q. What about seasonal variation?
    - Yes
    - Levels may be elevated in Winter #ClinicalPearl
- Q. How long can it be stored?

- In normal conditions, it can be stored easily
- Storage at 4 degrees is preferred for ion-exchange methods
- Long-term storage upto 10 years at -70 degrees is possible

- Q. Does drug intake interfere with the value?
  - Vitamin C and Aspirin in very high doses may have an impact
  - but are megadoses and not clinically relevant

- ***#ClinicalPearl- 50% of the value of HbA1c is impacted by the glucose value in the recent months time - so it is skewed mean and not exact mean of 3 months***

- Q. Does Iron deficiency anemia impact the HbA1c? #ClinicalPearl
  - Yes
  - it increases the HbA1c because of increased RBC lifespan
  - giving iron to these patients lowers the HbA1c

- Q. What happens to HbA1c in Sickle cell anemia?
  - HbA1c would not be accurate in Sickle-cell anemia
  - since SCA is associated with a defect in Beta-chain and HbA1c has to do with the beta-chain
  - Any form of Hemoglobinopathy that leads to lower or abnormal beta-chain leads to abnormality in HbA1c values

- Q. What HbA1c value can be useful for the diagnosis of Gestational Diabetes mellitus (GDM)? #ClinicalPearl
  - ***Ball-park figure- HBA1c of >5.9% strongly correlates with GDM***

- Q. Does hypothyroidism have any relation with HbA1c? #ClinicalPearl
  - Some studies have shown that Subclinical hypothyroidism and Overt hypothyroidism are associated with a mild increase of HbA1c which corrects on Levothyroxine supplementation

- Q. Is HbA1c reliable in a patient with cirrhosis? #ClinicalPearl
  - No
  - because of several factors HbA1c is not very reliable in patients with CLD

- Q. What about CKD? #ClinicalPearl
  - Some experts say
    - Don't use HBA1c for diagnosis of diabetes in CKD 1-3 - can use for monitoring therapy
    - Don't use HBA1c for diagnosis or treatment in patients with CKD 4/5 or ESRD

- Q. Which other drugs or factors can impact HbA1c?

- Dapsone significantly reduced HbA1c and hence HbA1c should not be used in patients receiving Dapsone
- Vitamin E may also reduce HBA1c levels
- Hydroxyurea may cause aberrant HbA1c levels

- Q. Why does Dapsone reduce the HbA1c?
  - By causing hemolysis
  - several antiretroviral drugs like Ribavarin also impact HbA1c in a similar way

- Q. Summarize the conditions producing false high and false low HBA1c.
  - Inappropriately Low HbA1c
    - - Hemolysis
    - - Certain hemoglobinopathies
    - - Recent blood transfusion
    - - Acute blood loss
    - - Hypertriglyceridemia
    - - Chronic liver disease
  - Inappropriately High HbA1c
    - - Iron deficiency
    - - Vitamin B12 deficiency
    - - Alcoholism
    - - Uremia
    - - Hyperbilirubinemia
  - Variable Effect on HbA1c+
    - - Fetal hemoglobin
    - - Methemoglobin
    - - Certain hemoglobinopathies

- Q. In which condition should you consider hemoglobinopathy and the aberrant result of HbA1c?
  i. HBA1c >15%
  ii. HBA1c and SMBG do not correlate
  iii. A dramatic difference in HBA1c based on change of lab or methodology

- Q. What is the impact of Hypertriglyceridemia on HbA1c?
  - It produces a false elevation of HbA1c
  - A similar thing is seen with glucocorticoid use

FIVE

HYPOGLYCEMIA IN PATIENTS WITH DIABETES MELLITUS

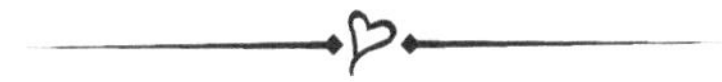

INTRODUCTION & DEFINITIONS

- Q. What are the symptoms of hypoglycemia?
  - Based on the Adrenergic system
    - Palpitations
    - Tremors
    - Anxiety
  - Based on the Cholinergic system
    - Hunger
    - Excessive sweating
    - Paraesthesia
  - Based on the Central nervous system
    - Seizures
    - Confusion
    - Abnormal behavior
    - Loss of consciousness
    - Fatigue
- Q. What is the difference between venous and arterial Blood glucose values?
  - Venous glucose is 20-30 mg/dl lower than arterial blood level in the fasting state
  - In postprandial – venous and arterial are the same
  - Whole blood is 10% lower than Plasma glucose
- Q. Why does hypoglycemia cause "Dead in bed syndrome"?

- Hypoglycemia may cause
    - QT prolongation
    - Increase QT dispersion
    - Increase the risk of arrhythmia
- Nocturnal hypoglycemia can cause arrhythmia in sleep dead in bed syndrome

- Q. What is the incidence of hypoglycemia in type 1 diabetics?
    - 1 episode per week
    - 1 severe hypoglycemia episode per year
- Q. What are the various categories of hypoglycemia in diabetics according to ADA?
    - Level 1 - Glucose between 54 - 70 mg/dl
    - Level 2- <54 mg/dl
    - Level 3- Any Hypoglycemia requiring assistance/ admission or altered sensorium etc
- Q. What is Probably symptomatic hypoglycemia?
    - Probably symptomatic hypoglycemia- symptoms present by BG not determined
- Q. What is relative hypoglycemia?
    - Relative hypoglycemia- symptoms of hypoglycemia but BG >70 mg/dl
- Q. What are the risk factors for hypoglycemia in diabetics?
    - Insulin–carbohydrate mismatch
    - Use of Sulphonylurea
    - Renal failure
    - Celiac disease
    - Liver failure
    - Exercise
    - Hypoglycemic unawareness / HAAF
    - Long-standing diabetes
    - Use of alcohol
    - Improved insulin sensitivity due to weight loss
- Q. Which Oral antidiabetics produce the highest risk of hypoglycemia?
    - Glibenclamide

HYPOGLYCEMIA-ASSOCIATED AUTONOMIC FAILURE

- Q. Which patients develop Hypoglycemia associated with autonomic failure (HAAF)?
    - Patients with diabetes with insulin deficiency
        - Long-standing Type 2 diabetes
        - Type 1 diabetes
- Q. What exactly happens in HAAF?
    - There is a loss of sympathoadrenal response to hypoglycemia
- Q. What is the mechanism of HAAF?

    i. Systemic mediator hypothesis

    - Hypoglycemia release some systemic mediator like Cortisol → which blunts response to subsequent hypoglycemia

    i. Brain fuel hypothesis

    - Hypoglycemia increases GLUT1 induction in the brain → normal glucose uptake in the brain despite low BG → hence the brain (hypothalamus) sympathoadrenal response does not occur
    - However, PET studies have refuted this hypothesis

    iii. Brain metabolism hypothesis

    - Hypoglycemia alters glucose metabolism in the brain → no response to hypoglycemia

    iv. Cerebral network hypothesis

    - The dorsal midline thalamus inhibits the Hypothalamus
    - Hypoglycemia→ activates dorsal midline thalamus
- Q. Is HAAF associated with autonomic neuropathy that occurs in diabetics?
    - No
    - It is a distinct syndrome NOT associated with autonomic neuropathy in diabetics
    - Autonomic neuropathy in diabetics also produces a similar picture but is a chronic process
- Q. What are the types of HAAF?
    - Sleep-related HAAF- diabetics are less aware of hypoglycemia during sleep unlike non-diabetics
    - Exercise-related HAAF nocturnal hypoglycemia occurs 6-8 hours after exercise
    - Antecedent HAAF → Previous hypoglycemia producing less response in subsequent hypoglycemia

- Q. How is HAAF treated?
    - It is treated by strict avoidance of hypoglycemia for 2-3 weeks corrects HAAF

PREVENTION OF HYPOGLYCEMIA IN PATIENTS WITH DIABETES

- Q. What are the three questions with regards to hypoglycemia that must be asked of a patient with diabetes in each visit?
    i. Any recorded episodes of hypoglycemia
    ii. Any symptoms suggestive of hypoglycemia
    iii. Episodes of hypoglycemia in which assistance of another individual was required (level 3 hypoglycemia)
- Q. What are the broad outlines for preventing hypoglycemia in patients with diabetes?
    i. Frequent SMBG
    ii. Patient Education
    iii. Rational treatment
    iv. Individualized HBA1c targets
    v. Identifying patients at higher risk
    vi. Diagnosis of Hypoglycemic unawareness and Autonomic neuropathy
- Q. Does technology help to reduce hypoglycemia?
    - Yes
    - CGM and Sensor augmented insulin pumps help to reduce the risk and severity of hypoglycemia
- Q. Does the use of an Insulin pump (CSII) itself reduce the risk of hypoglycemia?
    - No
    - The usual pumps do not reduce the risk of hypoglycemia
    - Sensor-augmented insulin pumps reduce the risk of hypoglycemia
- Q. What are the changes to the insulin that can be made to reduce hypoglycemia?
    - Use of newer basal insulin
    - Use of rapid-acting insulin analogs
- Q. What is done for patients with hypoglycemia unawareness?
    - 2-3 weeks of strict avoidance of hypoglycemia is helpful to restore awareness
    - Keep more lenient HBA1c goals in these patients
- Q. How much carbohydrate can be consumed by patients to prevent exercise-induced hypoglycemia?

  - 1 gram/kg/hour of carbohydrate intake

- Q. What is an option for patients with severe hypoglycemia with ESRD?
  - Pancreatic transplantation with kidney transplantation is a good option for these patients

ϷϷϷ

NOCTURNAL HYPOGLYCEMIA

- Q. What percentage of hypoglycemia observed in the DCCT trial was nocturnal?
  - 43%
- Q. What happens to the brain waves during hypoglycemia in an awake state?
  - there is a reduction in alpha waves but an increase in theta and delta waves
- Q. What happens in hypoglycemia during sleep?
  - In children- there are no changes in brain waves observed
  - In adults- when glucose is <45 mg/dl
    - There is a reduction of alpha waves
    - Prominent changes in theta waves
- Q. Does the brain have the same sensitivity to hypoglycemia during sleep, as when they are awake?
  - yes
  - The threshold for glucose values when brain wave changes occur suggests there is the same sensitivity for brain changes during sleep as it is during an awake state
  - Hence brain retains the inability to respond to hypoglycemia in sleep, at least in adults
- Q. But is the counter-regulatory response during sleep the same as during the awake state?
  - No
  - The counter-regulatory response to hypoglycemia is less profound during sleep than in an awake state
  - The glucagon response is preserved in non-diabetics, but in certain patients with diabetes it is blunted (see below)
  - The third line of defense, the sympathoadrenal response is reduced in people.
- Q. Does the stage of the sleep also determine the response?
  - Yes
  - The counter-regulatory response is also dependent on the stage of the sleep cycle when hypoglycemia occurs.

- Q. What is the clinical consequence on sleep quality in patients having nocturnal hypoglycemia?
    - Adults with recurrent nocturnal hypoglycemia have poor sleep quality
- Q. What percentage of nocturnal hypoglycemia is asymptomatic?
    - A large proportion are asymptomatic
        - 50% of adults and 78% of children are asymptomatic
        - It may even be prolonged and last for as much as 6 hours
- Q. What are the changes that occur to hepatic glucose production during sleep?
    - During sleep, hepatic glucose output reduces in response to reduced peripheral utilization of glucose
    - this is mainly driven by continuous basal insulin secretion
- Q. It is true that type 1 and type 2 diabetes with beta-cell failure have reduced counter-regulatory hormones also.
    - Yes
    - In type 1 diabetes and those with beta-cell failure in type 2 diabetes also have blunted glucagon response
    - This per se does not produce hypoglycemia but reduces their capacity to respond to hypoglycemia in case it develops
- Q. What are the Somogyi effect and the Dawn phenomenon?

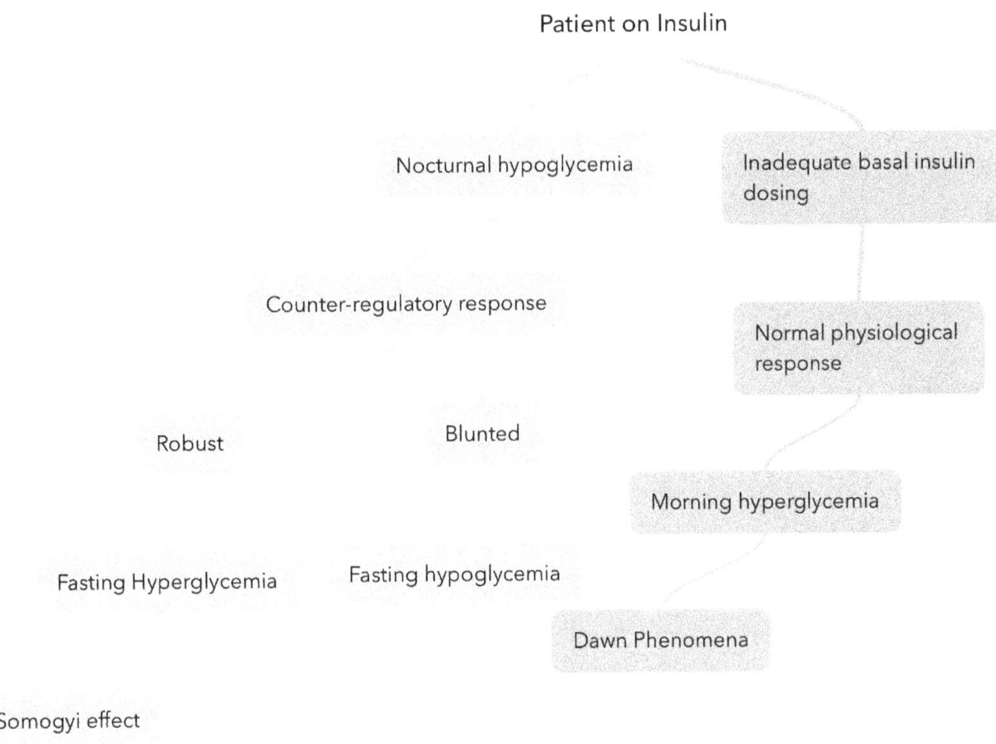

Figure 5.1: Somogyi Effect & Dawn Phenomenon

- Q. Does the Somogyi effect exist in reality?
    - Experimental evidence does show the existence of the Somogyi effect
    - However, even during the period of NPH insulin use, it was rare
    - The use of modern basal insulin nearly makes the phenomenon non-existent
- Q. What is a good reliable test for predicting the risk of nocturnal hypoglycemia?
    - The bedtime glucose value is a strong predictor of nocturnal hypoglycemia
    - Bedtime glucose associated with nocturnal hypoglycemia
        - <108 mg/dl in adults with type 1 diabetes
        - <130 mg/dl in children with type 1 diabetes
    - #Pearl:
        - Bedtime glucose is a good predictor of hypoglycemia earlier in the night
        - Fasting glucose a good predictor of early morning hypoglycemia

        - FBS <99 mg/dl for a patient on basal-bolus insulin suggests early morning hypoglycemia may have occurred

- Q. Which SMBG is useful for the diagnosis of nocturnal hypoglycemia?
    - 3 AM glucose reading
    - Though this is impractical
    - Hence CGM is useful for the diagnosis of nocturnal hypoglycemia
- Q. Broadly, what are the symptoms of nocturnal hypoglycemia?
    - Symptoms may be subtle and variable
        - Poor sleep quality
        - Vivid dreams and nightmares
        - Morning headache
        - Chronic fatigue
        - Mood changes
        - Night sweats and Wet bedsheets and bedclothes (because of sweat)
        - Enuresis (in children)
        - Restless behavior during sleep
- Q. Can it lead to mortality?
    - Yes
    - It can potentially trigger arrhythmia
    - The "Dead-in-the-bed" syndrome
    - Use of alcohol also contributes to the same in patients with diabetes
- Q. Can convulsions occur due to nocturnal hypoglycemia?
    - Yes
- Q. What are the long terms issues with nocturnal hypoglycemia?
    - Cognitive impairment
    - hypoglycemia unawareness
- Q. Can bedtime snacks reduce the risk of nocturnal hypoglycemia?
    - Yes
    - However, short-acting carbohydrates are not ideal for this purpose- they still make the patient vulnerable to hypoglycemia early in the morning
    - Uncooked cornstarch is ideal for such an action
    - Adding acarbose before dinner is also a useful way of preventing nocturnal hypoglycemia in both type 1 and type 2 diabetes
- Q. What are the other ways of preventing nocturnal hypoglycemia?

i. Using modern long-acting basal insulin analogs

- Glargine U300
- Insulin degludec

i. Using rapidly acting insulin analogs before dinner
ii. Use of sensor-augmented insulin pumps

- Q. Does giving glargine U100 in the morning reduce the risk of nocturnal hypoglycemia?
  - Yes
  - In some patients, this is seen
  - This is probably because glargine U100 may not work for 24 hours in some patients- hence the effect of glargine wears off during nighttime
  - However, insulin glargine U300 solves this problem

ÞÞÞ

SULPHONYLUREA INDUCED HYPOGLYCEMIA

- Q. How are Sulphonylurea metabolised?
  - They are metabolised via the liver and have active metabolites excreted via the kidney
  - hence both liver dysfunction and renal dysfunction can cause Sulphonylurea hypoglycemia
  - They are also protein-bound and hence have a longer half-life
- Q. Which are the most common neuroglycopenic symptoms of hypoglycemia?
  - Confusion
  - Personality change
- Q. Which are the most common autonomic symptoms of hypoglycemia?
  - Diaphoresis
  - Tremors
- Q. What kind of hypoglycemia is caused by Sulphonylurea?
  - insulin-dependent hypoglycemia
  - Elevated insulin and c-peptide levels in the presence of hypoglycemia is a critical sample
- Q. How is hypoglycemia acutely corrected with IV Dextrose?
  - Adults- 1-2ml/kg (generally 25 gram- 50ml) of 50% dextrose
  - Children - 2-4 ml/kg of 25% dextrose
  - Infant- 5-10 ml/kg of 10% dextrose

    - Once the acute correction is given - continuous glucose infusion is continued

- Q. Which other vitamin must be given with dextrose?

    - If Thiamine deficiency is suspected- give 100 mg IV of thiamine along with the glucose
    - This is to prevent Wernicke's encephalopathy

- Q. Can glucagon be given in this setting?

    - Yes
    - But this is not a substitute for IV Dextrose

- Q. What is done in case of a symptomatic intentional overdose of Sulphonylurea?

    - this must be treated with both IV Dextrose and Octreotide
    - IV dextrose- though important must not be used alone
    - this is because IV dextrose can lead to hyperglycemia → which stimulates the release of insulin further
    - Hence Octreotide must be given along with IV dextrose
    - Octreotide blocks the further release of insulin
    - A continuous IV Dextrose infusion may also be given

- Q. How is Octreotide given?

    - it is given in the dose of 50-100 mcg subcutaneously or IM every 6 hours in adults.
    - In children, it is given 1-1.5 mcg/kg every 6 hrly
    - It can also be given as IV infusion, but subcutaneous or IM is enough in most cases

- Q. How long is Octreotide given?

    - It is given for 24 hours
    - generally not required to repeat after the same
    - If hypoglycemia persists after 24 hours- then repeat Octreotide

- Q. How is IV dextrose infusion given?

    - Adults 5% dextrose - 75-100 ml/hr
    - Children- 6-9 mg/kg/min dextrose infusion

- Q. How is a rate of infusion calculated based on mg/kg/min?

    - Rate of Infusion = (dose required in mg/kg/min x 6 x weight) / Percent dextrose in solution
    - for example 10 kg child, needing 8 mg/kg/min infusion of 10% dextrose- give 48 ml/hr based on the above calculation

- Q. Apart from Octreotide which other medication can be used?

    - Diazoxide
    - But Octreotide is better than Diazoxide

- Q. Is Octreotide also given during a single episode of level 2 or level 3 Sulphonylurea-induced hypoglycemia?
    - No
    - Octreotide is not required for a single episode of Sulphonylurea induced hypoglycemia
    - It is to be given only when there is level 3 hypoglycemia, intentional overdose, or multiple episodes of level 2 hypoglycemia
    - In a single episode- observe the patient for 24 hours- if there is a second episode then give Octreotide else discharge after 24 hours of observation
    - IV dextrose may be given as appropriate and carbohydrate-rich meal may be given

NEWER UPDATES

- Q. What are ADIPs ?
    - Algorithm-driven insulin pumps
    - 1/ Algorithm-driven insulin pumps, also known as "smart pumps" or "artificial pancreas systems", use mathematical algorithms to adjust insulin delivery in real-time.
    - 2/ These pumps include a continuous glucose monitor (CGM) that measures glucose levels and a pump that delivers insulin.
    - 3/ The algorithm uses the glucose data from the CGM to calculate the appropriate insulin dose and adjust the pump accordingly.
    - 4/ Examples of algorithm-driven insulin pumps include Medtronic MiniMed 670G, 780G and Tandem t:slim X2 insulin pump.
    - 5/ These pumps are designed to reduce the burden of diabetes management by automatically adjusting insulin delivery and can help reduce the risk of hypoglycemia and hyperglycemia and improve overall diabetes control.
    - 6/ Overall, Algorithm-driven insulin pumps are becoming increasingly popular among people with diabetes, as they can provide a more effective and efficient way to manage the disease.
- Q. For patients with type 1 diabetes- should SMBG be used regularly or should CGM be used regularly?
    - The new guidelines suggest the use of CGM rather than SMBG in patients with Type 1 Diabetes
    - SMBG can be used to confirm the abnormal glucose readings from CGM
- Q. What about pumps?
    - The guidelines recommend the use of ADIPs for patients with type 1 diabetes to reduce the burden of hypoglycemia
- Q. Can we use CGM for Hospital hyperglycemia?
    - Yes
    - Current guidelines recommend the use of CGM in selected patients for Hospital hyperglycemia to prevent hypoglycemia episodes
    - This is provided that extremes of glucose values are cross-checked with glucometers

- Q. In which patients is CGM recommended for Hospital hyperglycemia?
- Q. In which hospitalized patient can you expect inaccurate readings with CGM ?
    - Extensive skin infection
    - Hypoperfusion
    - Hypovolumeia
    - Medications
        - Inotrope use
        - Those on acetaminophen > 4 grams/day
        - Dopamine
        - Vitamin C
        - Heparin
        - Hydroxyurea

References

1. McCall AL, Lieb DC, Gianchandani R, MacMaster H, Maynard GA, Murad MH, Seaquist E, Wolfsdorf JI, Wright RF, Wiercioch W. Management of Individuals With Diabetes at High Risk for Hypoglycemia: An Endocrine Society Clinical Practice Guideline. The Journal of Clinical Endocrinology & Metabolism. 2022 Dec 7.
2. Allen KV, Frier BM. Nocturnal hypoglycemia: clinical manifestations and therapeutic strategies toward prevention. Endocr Pract. 2003 Nov-Dec;9(6):530-43. doi: 10.4158/EP.9.6.530. PMID: 14715482.

SIX

PATHOGENESIS OF TYPE 2 DIABETES IN INDIAN POPULATION

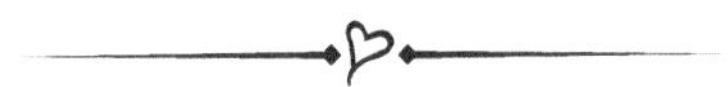

- Q. What are the three key features of type 2 diabetes in Indian and Chinese populations?

    i. Younger age at diagnosis
    ii. More beta-cell failure
    iii. Leaner body habitus

- Q. What pathophysiological feature is seen in first-degree relatives of patients with type 2 diabetes that determines that there is probably a genetic component to diabetes?

    - Relatives of patients with type 2 diabetes have impaired first-phase and second-phase insulin secretion compared to other normal population
    - this may predispose them to develop type 2 diabetes in the future

- Q. What is the key pathophysiological driver in patients with type 2 diabetes of South Asian origin and what studies have validated this?

    - The British Whitehall study, the MASALA, and the MESA studies looked at the pathophysiological differences in South Asians versus Europeans
    - They found that the HOMA-S was lower in South Asians compared to Europeans but in both cases declined with age
    - The HOMA-Beta- representing insulin response peaked 15 years earlier in South Asians and declined earlier compared to Europeans suggesting early exhaustion of compensatory mechanisms in South Asians compared to Caucasians
    - This tells us that Beta-cell dysfunction occurs earlier in Indian patients with type 2 diabetes compared to Europeans

- Q. Apart from HOMA-Beta, what are the other methods by which you can determine the decline in beta-cell function over a period of time?

    i. Oral disposition index

ii. Glycemic deterioration over time - as evidenced by slipe of HbA1c over time

- Q. What is the formulation for Oral disposition index?
  - Oral disposition index = Insulin sensitivity index (Matsuda index) x insulin secretion index
    - Insulin sensitivity index = ISI = 10,000/square root of (Insulin at fasting × Glucose at fasting) × (mean glucose × mean insulin during OGTT) ==> note 75-g oral glucose test is used and blood samples were taken at 0, 30, 60, 90, and 120 min for the measurement of plasma glucose and insulin concentrations
    - Insulin secreation index = ΔI30/ΔG30 = (Ins30-Ins0)/(Glu30-Glu0)
      - Insulin and glucose at 30 minutes and baseline
- Q. In Indian patients with prediabetes- is there more IFG or more IGT?
  - There is more IFG compared to IGT
  - This is similar to non-caucasian cohorts in the US
  - The increase in IFG represents hepatic insulin resistance
  - HOMA-IR correlates well with hepatic insulin resistance
- Q. What is the distinct difference in the insulin resistance patterns in Indian versus the Chinese?
  - The Chinese have more Skeletal muscle insulin resistance and Indians have more hepatic insulin resistance
  - Hence Chinese Pre-diabetics have more IGT while Indians have more IFG
- Q. Which are the distinct alleles found from the GWAS study in the UK biobank in the Indian population that predispose them to develop Type 2 Diabetes?
  - HNF4A - Deals with insulin secretion
  - GRB14- deals with the action of insulin receptor
  - ST6GAL1- deals with insulin action
  - TMEM163- associated with insulin secretion
- Q. What are the broad interpretations of the UK biobank studies?
  i. Indians tend to have more issues with insulin secretion
  ii. The alleles for subcutaneous adiposity are missing- hence Indians tend to have visceral adiposity
- Q. What are the common histopathological features seen in Indian and Chinese type 2 diabetes patients?
  - Islet amyloid deposits in the pancreas are common in Indian and Chinese populations
  - They are seen in 40-100% of the patients
- Q. Summarize the key points in the pathogenesis of type 2 diabetes in Indians.

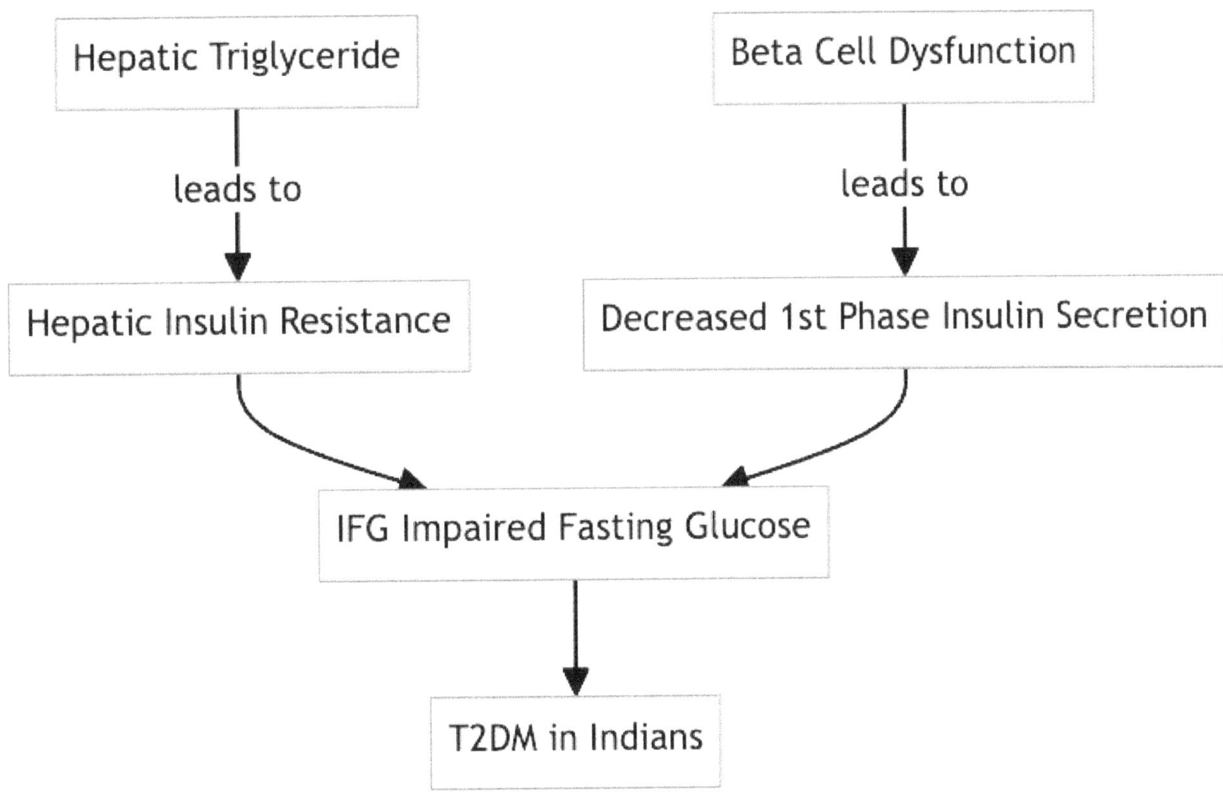

Figure 6.1 : Key points in the pathogenesis of Type 2 Diabetes in Indians

- Q. What is the ANDIS classification of Diabetes mellitus?
  - Tags: Diabetes classification; Swedish cluster; Subtype of Diabetes; ANDIS classification
  - This is the classification of diabetes from the Swedish Cluster
  - SAID = Severe Autoimmune Diabetes
    - GAD antibodies, low insulin secretion, poor metabolic control
  - SIDD = Severe Insulin Deficient Diabetes
    - Low insulin secretion, poor metabolic control, increased risk of retinopathy
  - SIRD = Severe Insulin Resistant Diabetes
    - Insulin resistance, obesity, late-onset, marked increased risk of nephropathy
  - MOD = Moderate Obesity-Related Diabetes

        - Obesity, early-onset, good metabolic control
    - MARD = Moderate Age-Related Diabetes
        - Late-onset, good metabolic control, low risk of complications
- Q. What is the frequency of these clusters in the Indian cohorts?
    - The data from this comes from the INSPIRED and INDIAB studies
    - The frequencies are as follows:

    i. Severe insulin-deficient diabetes- 26-27%
    ii. Severe insulin-resistant diabetes-7-12%
    iii. Moderate obesity-related diabetes- 25-30%
    iv. Mild age-related diabetes- 34-35%

- Q. What were the features of the Severe insulin-deficient diabetes cluster in the Indian population?

    i. It was more often compared to the Swedish (26% vs 17%)
    ii. At younger age (42 vs 57 years)
    iii. Lower BMI
    iv. Lower beta-cell function
    v. lower insulin resistance

    b. Interestingly even the severe insulin-resistant cluster of Indian patients had lower HOMA-Beta values (meaning more beta-cell dysfunction) compared to the Swedish cohort

- Q. Is the beta-cell decline in Young diabetics faster compared to others?
    - Yes
    - Type 2 diabetes before age of 40 years as studied in the TODAY trial showed more rapid deterioration of beta-cell function
    - this was evidenced by a rapidly declining oral disposition index at rate of 20-30% per year
- Q. Why are DPP-4 inhibitors more effective in the Indian population?
    - they say that it restores First phase insulin secreation earlier
    - hence more effective
- Q. What are the special issues with Thiazolidinones in the Asian population?
    - It seems that in the Asian population- the increased risk for heart failure hospitalization is not seen with these class of drugs
    - Tags: Pioglitazone
- Q. What are the summary and conclusion of this article?

i. The age of onset of diabetes in the Indian population may be younger compared to the west. Diabetes before 40 years of age is very common
ii. Indian cohorts tend to have lower beta-cell function compared to the western cohorts. This is the key pathophysiological point and must always be kept in mind
iii. Severe insulin-deficient diabetes is a common cluster in the Indian subset of patients
iv. Overall, Indian diabetes is leaner, and subcutaneous fat deposition is lesser
v. Incretin-based therapies and AGI tend to do very well in the Indian subset of patients, especially when initiated when beta-cells are well-preserved

Reference :

1. Ke, C., Narayan, K.M., Chan, J.C., Jha, P. and Shah, B.R., 2022. Pathophysiology, phenotypes, and management of type 2 diabetes mellitus in Indian and Chinese populations. **Nature Reviews Endocrinology**, pp.1-20

SEVEN

BLOOD GLUCOSE MONITORING & GLUCOMETERS

Q. What precautions are taken while drawing plasma blood glucose?

- Collect from arm different from where IV line is to avoid contamination with IV fluid
- Centrifuge and ship in Ice or use fluoride bulb

Q. Which is higher – whole glucose values or plasma glucose values?

- Plasma glucose values are higher than whole glucose values by 12-15%

Q. What is the difference between venous and arterial blood glucose?

- In fasting – Venous and arterial are the same
- Post-meal- venous are less than arterial by 10%

Q. What is the SI unit for glucose?

- Mmol/liter
- To convert to mg/dl – multiply by 18

Q. Which are the two major ways in which blood glucose is measured?

- Glucose oxidase methods – GOD/POD
- Enzymatic method

Q. Which of the above is better?

- Enzymatic method is more sensitive and specific
- Glucose oxidase methods are cheaper

Q. Which is the reference enzymatic method?

- Hexokinase/G6PDH method

Q. Which substances in the blood produce an error with GOD /POD?

- Reducing substances
- Ascorbic acid
- Tetracycline
- Glutathione
- Bilirubin

Q. Describe the enzymatic reaction in the GOD-POD method?

- Glucose + O_2 → (Via Glucose oxidase Enzyme) → Glucuronic acid + H_2O_2
- H_2O_2+ Reduced dye = H_2O + Oxidized dye
- Oxidized dye is measured
- H_2O_2 can also be monitored electrochemically

Q. What type of glucose does Glucose oxidase act upon?

- Acts upon beta D glucose and does not act on alpha D glucose
- This is a very specific step in GOD-POD

Q. Give the chemical reaction for Hexokinase / G6PDH method?

- Glucose → (hexokinase enzyme) → Glucose-6 phosphate + ADP
- Glucose – 6 phosphate → (G6PDH enzyme) → 6 phosphogluconate + NADPH + H
- NADPH is measured using fluorescence

Q. What method is used in most labs?

- Glucose oxidase method on Beckman Coulter Unicel DXC-800 analyzer

Q. What blood glucose values are reported by glucometers compared to the laboratory?

- Glucometers report whole blood glucose values
- While Labs report plasma glucose
- However, most modern glucometers now display the glucose value corrected to the plasma glucose value

Q. What are the ISO standards for glucometers?

- Blood glucose <70 mg/dl- 95% of reading should be within 15 mg/dl
- Blood glucose > 70 mg/dl- should be within 20%

Q. What is the purpose of fluoride bulbs, and what does it inhibit?

- RBC in the blood utilize the glucose for energy by glycolysis
- Hence the glucose values reduce during transport
- Hence, fluoride inhibits the enolase enzyme, which prevents the glycolysis during transport

Q. How long is it stable at room temperature with a fluoride bulb?

- 72 hours at room temperature in fluoride bulb

Q. How long is it stable when serum is separate, and fluoride is not used?

- 8 hours at 25 degree
- 72 hours at 4 degree

Q. If heparin is used to separate the plasma- what is the difference in values?

- Glucose value is 5% lower if heparin is used

Q. Is finger prick glucose – arterial or venous?

- It is arterial

Q. Which part of the finger is the prick done and why?

- Lateral aspect of the fingertip
- This has fewer nerve endings
- Hence it reduces the pain

Q. What is the typical range for blood glucose strips?

- 10-600 mg/dl

Q., if glucometer strips are cut in half, will it reduce its accuracy?

- No

Q. How do the glucometers measure the reading?

- They use one of the two methods
- Reflectance photometry- a reflection of light by the chromogen product obtained by glucose oxidase method
- Amperometric method- measures the electric current generated by the glucose oxidase method
- Reflectance photometry is better

Q. How does hematocrit affect the glucose values?

- When BG >300 mg/dl- hematocrit >55% can lower the BG value by 15%, likewise the hematocrit <35 % can increase the BG value by 10%

Q. What methods for glucose testing are utilized by most glucometer strips?

- 1. Glucose oxidase method
- 2. Hexokinase/G6PDH method (Glucose dehydrogenase-nicotinamide dinucleotide)
- 3. GDH-Flavin adenine dinucleotide
- 4. GDH-PQQ - glucose dehydrogenase pyrroloquinoline quinone (GDH-PQQ) glucose test strips

Q. Of these above methods, which one is most likely to give false results due to interference?

- GDH-PQQ method
- This method is not specific to glucose
- Apart from glucose, it also catalyzes other sugars like maltose, galactose, and xylose

Q. How does Vitamin C lead to interference with the glucometer values?

- Vitamin C mainly produces interference with the GDH-PQQ method
- This is because vitamin C is an antioxidant
- it inactivates free radical and itself if oxidised on the surface of the strip to produce electrons which produce the current by the Amperometric method
- This produces false high values

Q. Which other common substances can produce similar interferences?

- Maltose producing substances
- Icodextrin present in peritoneal fluid
- Certain immunoglobulins like abatacept, tositumomab, etc

Q. Which common glucometers use the GDH-PQQ method?

- ACCU-CHEK by Roche
- FreeStyle by Abbott Diabetes Care

Q. Has FDA given a warning for the GDH-PQQ?

- Yes
- FDA has issued a warning for the same

Q. Does the ACCU-CHECK available in India also have the GDH-PQQ method?

- No. It uses the Mut Q-GDH method

Q. Enlist the interfering substances with various glucometers as suggested by ADA guidelines 2021?

- Glucose oxidase monitors
- Uric acid
- Galactose
- Xylose
- Acetaminophen
- L-DOPA
- Ascorbic acid
- Glucose dehydrogenase monitors
- Icodextrin (used in peritoneal dialysis)

Q. Give the FDA mandated standards for blood glucose monitors?

- Home use:

  - - 95% within 15% for all BG in the usable BG range
  - - 99% within 20% for all BG in the usable BG range

- Hospital use:

  - - 95% within 12% for BG ≥75 mg/dL
  - - 95% within 12 mg/dL for BG <75 mg/dL
  - - 98% within 15% for BG ≥75 mg/dL
  - - 98% within 15 mg/dL for BG <75 mg/dL

Q. What is the impact of oxygen levels on Glucometers ?

- Glucometers that use glucose oxidase method are more likely to be impacted by oxygen levels
- Glucose dehydrogenase method glucometers are NOT impacted by oxygen levels
- Higher oxygen tensions- arterial blood or oxygen therapy may result in false low values
- Lower oxygen tensions - can cause false high readings
- High altitude
- Hypoxia
- Venous blood readings

EIGHT

METFORMIN IN PREGNANCY

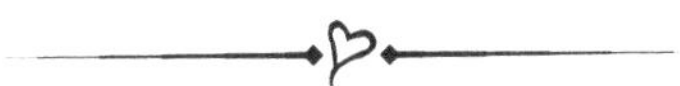

Q. What is the rationale for the use of metformin in pregnancy?

- 1. Treatment of Gestational Diabetes mellitus (GDM)
- 2. Treatment of pregestational diabetes
- 3. Patients on PCOS becoming pregnant- 4. Gestational obesity

Q. What is the category for metformin in pregnancy?

- Metformin is in pregnancy category B
- This is the same as insulin
- Category B is defined as
- "Either animal-reproduction studies have not demonstrated a fetal risk, but there are no controlled studies in pregnant women or animal-reproduction studies have shown an adverse effect (other than a decrease in fertility) that was not confirmed in controlled studies in women in the first trimester (and there is no evidence of a risk in later trimesters)."

Q. Does first-trimester exposure to metformin produce congenital abnormalities?

- No
- A case-control study by Given et al. found no congenital abnormalities
- There was the chance finding of increased pulmonary atresia, but this was more likely to be a chance finding - "No evidence was found for an increased risk of all nongenetic congenital anomalies combined following exposure to metformin during the first trimester, and the one significant association was no more than would be expected by chance. Further surveillance is needed to increase sample size and follow up the cardiac signal, but these findings are reassuring given the increasing use of metformin in pregnancy" [1]

Q. Can metformin be used in the management of gestational obesity?

- Rationale- metformin can potentially prevent maternal weight gain and reduce the risk of GDM in pregnancy - RCT has shown that metformin does prevent maternal weight gain
- Reduces risk of preeclampsia
- Also reduces the risk of neonatal ICU admission
- However, it does not prevent GDM
- It also does not reduce the risk for large gestational age babies

USE OF METFORMIN IN PREGESTATIONAL DIABETES

Q. What is the MITY study?

- This is the study done to see the effect of metformin in women with type 2 diabetes and pregnancy
- This is an RCT
- Women were already on insulin
- Women were randomized to receive metformin 1 gram BDversus placebo added to insulin
- The results were encouraging
- The study found better glycemic control with the use of metformin and less large for gestational age infants
- However, the risk of small for gestational age was increased

Q. Overall, what is the understanding of metformin with regard to the size of infants?

- Clearly, metformin produces smaller infants
- But there might for a post-natal growth acceleration leading large children at a later date

Q. Which guidelines support the use of metformin for hyperglycemia in pregnancy?

- 1. NICE guidelines
- 2. Society for Maternal-fetal medicine

Q. What are the benefits of the use of metformin in hyperglycemia in pregnancy?

- 1. Less pregnancy weight gain
- 2. Less hypoglycemia
- 3. Better patient acceptability
- 4. Reduces risk of preeclampsia
- 5. Reduces risk of preterm delivery

Q. What are the benefits of metformin over insulin in hyperglycemia in pregnancy?

- 1. Lower Large for Gestational age babies
- 2. Less neonatal hypoglycemia
- 3. Less neonatal ICU admission

Q. What are the biggest challenge with the use of Metformin in pregnancy?

- 1. High rate of ineffectiveness as a form of treatment for
    - Hyperglycemia in pregnancy
    - 46% of women on metformin required insulin (Rowan et al.2008)
- 2. Metformin does cross the placenta (however, it does not seem to have any adverse fetal effects) - 3. Long term impact is NOT known

Q. Is metformin in pregnancy safe?

- Yes
- Conclusion for meta-analysis of 6 RCTs have concluded that the use for metformin in pregnancy is safe

Q. Is metformin use in the first trimester of pregnancy associated with an increased risk of fetal teratogenicity?

- No
- Several studies and meta-analyses have been reassuring of this

Q. What are the issues with PCOS women becoming pregnant?

- The odds of several complications in pregnancy are more women having PCOS compared to normal women - This makes continuing metformin in these women an attractive option

Q. Does continuing or starting metformin in women with PCOS have any benefit?

- The conclusion comes from an RCT by Vanky et al
- They found
- No effect of prevention of GDM in these women with metformin use (some other studies have shown that it does prevent GDM)
- The main benefit was a reduction of preterm delivery- This is in contrast to other situations where the use of metformin is associated with higher preterm birth

Q. What are the long-term impact of the use of Metformin in pregnancy when used in the context of Hyperglycemia in pregnancy?

- 18 months
    - Children exposed to metformin are taller and heavier compared to their counterparts not exposed to metformin
    - No neurodevelopmental issues
- 2 years
    - Large skinfold thickness in children exposed to metformin in fetal life
    - But DEXA did not show a difference in fat percentage
- 9 Years
    - meta-analysis clearly shows that in utero exposure leads to heavier and taller children - Also, DEXA fat mass is more
    - Hence since they are heavier and taller, the BMI Z-scores were not different compared to the control - The main data from this meta-analysis comes from the MIG-TOFU study

Q. Is metformin secreted in breast milk?

- Yes

Q. What is the MiG trial?

- This is the most important trial comparing the use of metformin and insulin in GDM patients
- 46% of patients on metformin did require insulin- However, the composite endpoint of perinatal outcomes was the same in the metformin and the insulin group - There was no adverse effect with the use of metformin - 70% of the women preferred using metformin over insulin

METFORMIN IN PREGNANCY - SUMMARY, AND CONCLUSIONS

- 1. Treatment of Gestational Diabetes mellitus (GDM)
- Use insulin as the first line of therapy
- Metformin can be added to therapy
- this is as per the guidelines
- MiG trial may be useful here
- 2. Treatment of pregestational diabetes
- MITY study
- Found benefit of using Insulin + metformin versus insulin + placebo
- Must be used
- 3. Patients with PCOS becoming pregnant
- Venky et al. found no major benefit for the prevention of GDM and other parameters
- In some parameters, it was useful
- Can be used till the end of the first trimester then stopped
- 4. Gestational obesity
- There is no indication of use
- Does not prevent GDM
- No major benefit
- Don't use

ppp

References:

1. Given JE, Loane M, Garne E, Addor MC, Bakker M, BertautNativel B, Gatt M, Klungsoyr K, Lelong N, Morgan M, Neville AJ. Metformin exposure in first trimester of pregnancy and risk of all or specific congenital anomalies: exploratory case-control study.

NINE

C-PEPTIDE

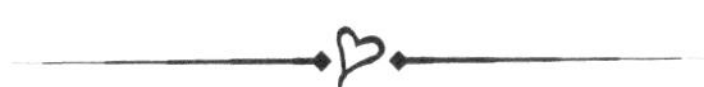

- Q. What is C-peptide ?
    - The pancreatic proinsulin is broken down into insulin and C-peptide
    - The C-peptide is released in equimolar concentration as insulin
- Q. What are the various ways in which C-peptide is measured?
    - C peptide measurement in blood
        - Fasting
        - Stimulated
        - Random C peptide
    - Urine C peptide can also be measured – requires 24-hour collection
- Q. Of the above, which is a good marker of Beta-cell reserve?
    - Stimulated C peptide is a marker of Beta cell reserve
- Q. What are the methods for "stimulation" in C-peptide?
    - Glucose load
    - Mixed meal
    - Glucagon
- Q. Broadly, what is the difference between C-peptide in type 1 and type 2 diabetes in terms of stimulation test?
    - Type 1 there is little or no increase in C peptide over baseline
    - Type 2 there is some increase in C peptide over baseline
- Q. What basal c-peptide value helps discriminate type 1 from type 2 diabetes?
    - About 80% of Basal C-peptide levels below a cutoff of 0.6 ng/ml (0.2 nmol/l) have type 1 diabetes
    - Similarly, 80% of patients with stimulated C-peptide <1 nmol/l have type 1 diabetes

- Q. Is Random C-peptide useful?
    - One study showed that random C peptide was better than fasting and stimulated C peptide for the classification of diabetes mellitus
- Q. What is the interpretation of non-fasting Random c-peptide value ?
    - <0.6 ng/ml - Strongly suggestive of absolute insulin deficiency and type 1 diabetes
    - <1.8 ng/ml- Unlikely to achieve glycemic control without the use of Multiple insulin doses
    - More than 3 ng/ml- Unlikely to be type 1 diabetes- more likely to be Type 2 or MODY
- Q. Describe the protocol for glucagon-stimulated C-peptide
    - Draw baseline fasting specimen. (12 hours of overnight fast)
    - Administer 1 mg Glucagon I.V.
    - Draw additional specimens at 6 and 10 minutes post-glucagon
- Q. What is the protocol for the mixed-meal stimulation test?
    i. Fasting - Measure FBS and C-peptide
    ii. Give liquid mixed meal - Sustacal or Ensure Plus powder - 6 scoops in 200 ml water
    iii. Measure RBS and C-peptide 90 min after liquid meals
- Q. What is Sustacal ?
    - It is a protein supplement from Nestle
    - ENSURE PLUS powder can be used as a substitute which has a similar composition
- Q. In terms of percentage what is the percentage of C-peptide elevation post-baseline
    - Normal stimulation of c-peptide is a 150-300% elevation over basal levels.
- Q. Give the scoring of C-peptide post-mixed meal stimulation used by the Department of Endocrinology at Zydus Hospital? (Unpublished)

Fasting/Post-stimulation	Value of C-peptide	Grading	Points
FASTING	<0.24 ng/ml	Grade 1F	Score 5
FASTING	0.24-0.6 ng/ml	Grade 2F	Score 3
FASTING	0.6-1 ng/ml	Grade 3F	Score 1
FASTING	More than 1 ng/ml	Grade 4F	Score 0
POST STIMULATION / RANDOM	<0.6 ng/ml	Grade 1S	Score 5
POST STIMULATION / RANDOM	0.6-1.5 ng/ml	Grade 2S	Score 3
POST STIMULATION / RANDOM	1.5-1.8 ng/ml-	Grade 3S	Score 2
POST STIMULATION / RANDOM	1.8-3.3 ng/ml	Grade 4S	Score 1
POST STIMULATION / RANDOM	More than 3.3 ng/ml	Grade 5S	Score 0

Table 9.1: Mixed meal stimulation test scoring

- Total score
    - ≥5 - strongly suggestive of Type 1 diabetes
    - 3-5- Suggestive of type 1
    - 0-3- Unlikely to be type 1 but close follow-up is required
    - 0 - not type 1

- Q. In a patient with type 2 diabetes, what value of C peptide suggests the need for basal-bolus insulin (Multiple dose insulin) for diabetes management as compared to basal insulin with OAD?
    - Post-stimulation C-peptide <3.1 ng/ml - suggestive of the need for MDI therapy instead of basal-only
- Q. What cut-off is suggestive of Insulin-mediated hypoglycemia in patients undergoing a 72-hour fast test for hypoglycemia evaluation?
    - When the glucose value is <55 mg/dl- a C-peptide value of >0.6 ng/ml is strongly suggestive of insulin-mediated hypoglycemia

TEN

FIBROCALCULOUS PANCREATIC DIABETES (FCPD)

- Q. What is the definition of Fibrocalculous pancreatic diabetes (FCPD)?
    - Diabetes associated with non-alcoholic calcific pancreatitis seen in developing countries
- Q. What is the prediabetic form of FCPD?
    - It is called tropical calcific pancreatitis (TCP)
- Q. Give the difference between TCP and Alcoholic pancreatitis.

	TCP	Alcoholic pancreatitis
Age of onset	20-30 years	30-50 years
Sex M:F	70:30	90:10
Alcohol abuse	absent	Present
Dilated ducts	present	Absent
Diabetes	90%	50%
Calcification	In large ducts	In small ducts
Risk of pancreatic cancer	Very high	increased
calculi	90%	50%
fibrosis	heavy	Present

Table 10.1: Difference between TCP and Alcoholic pancreatitis

- Q. Who is the father of FCPD?

    - Geeverghese

- Q. Which are the two types of malnutrition-related DM (MRDM)?
    - Fibrocalculous pancreatic diabetes
    - Protein-deficient diabetes mellitus
- Q. What is the typical triad of FCPD?
    - Abdominal pain- the first symptom- in childhood
    - Pancreatic calculi- In adolescent
    - Diabetes in adulthood
- Q. Where is the calcification seen in Plain Xray in FCPD?
    - Close to L1/L2 vertebra
- Q. Ketosis is present in FCPD. True or false?
    - False
    - Patients with FCPD do not develop ketosis
- Q. Intake of which food substance is implicated in causing FCPD?
    - Cassava
- Q. Which cancer risk is increased in FCPD?
    - Pancreatic cancer
- Q. There are no microvascular complications in FCPD, True or false?
    - False
    - It was believed earlier but not so anymore
    - Microvascular complications are very much present in patients with FCPD
- Q. What are the diagnostic criteria for FCPD?
    - As given by Mohan et al
        - Essential criteria
            - Diabetes present
            - A patient from a tropical country
            - Absence of any other cause of pancreatitis
    - Any 3 of the following

    - Abnormal morphology of pancreas on imaging
    - Abnormal pancreatic function test
    - Abdominal pain recurrent since childhood
    - Steatorrhea

- Q. Which is the tumor marker for pancreatic cancer?
  - CA 19-9

- Q. What is the classical clinical description of a patient with FCPD?
  - Cyanotic hue
  - emaciated
  - Parotidomegaly
  - Abdominal distension

- Q. Why is there no ketosis in FCPD?
  - Some of the theories for the absence of ketosis in FCPD are as follows
    - No non-esterified fatty acid hence less substrate for ketosis
    - Also, there is reduced glucagon along with insulin
      - High glucagon and reduced insulin are required for ketosis to develop
    - The fat present is resistant to lipolysis
    - There is some residual beta-cell function
    - Carnitine deficiency prevents Fatty acid from entering the mitochondria for beta-oxidation

- Q. Is the calcification present in the parenchyma or in the duct?
  - FCPD- in the duct
  - Alcoholic pancreatitis in the parenchyma

- Q. What is the composition of the calculi?
  - It is composed of calcium carbonate

- Q. Can ERCP and EUS be used to define pancreatic morphology in FCPD?
  - Yes

- Q. Which is the invasive test for detecting pancreatic function?
  - Injection of secretin and Pancreozymin
  - Collection of pancreatic juice
  - Juice contains less lipase, bicarbonate, and trypsin compared to normal

- Q. Which are non-invasive (tubeless tests for pancreatic function) ?
  - BT-PABA (Bentriomide para aminobenzyoic acid) - Urine / plasma
  - Fecal elastase
  - Fecal chymotrypsin
- Q. Which is the gold standard Tubeless test?
  - Fecal elastase
- Q. How Is endocrine pancreatic function tested for in FCPD?
  - Using C-peptide
  - The value is intermediate between type 1 and type 2 suggestive of residual pancreatic function
- Q. What is done for abdominal pain in FCPD?
  - It occurs earlier
  - Non-opiod / opiod analgesisc are used
  - It resolves once the endocrine dysfunction occurs
  - Pancreatic enzyme supplementation does not reduce the pain
- Q. What is done for non resolving pain ?
  - ESWL + ERCP
  - Celiac plexus block
  - Surgery drainage procedures ductal decompression or pancreaticojejunostomy
  - Surgery ablative procedures partial or subtotal pancreatectomy
- Q. What is done for the management of steatorrhea?
  - Pancreatic enzyme supplementation
  - Reduce diet fat
  - Give vitamins
- Q. What is the dose of pancreatic enzyme supplementation in these patients?
  - The typical brand name is "Creon" 10,000 units before each meal

In clinical practice is is observed that giving pancreatic enzyme supplement also has some beneficial effect on glycemic control. Some experts have suggested a link between the exocrine and endocrine dysfunctions.

- Q. What is the best treatment for diabetes in these patients?
  - 85% require insulin

- Some may do well with OAD because of residual pancreatic function
- However, incretin-based therapies are best avoided
- They often have brittle diabetes and are prone to hypoglycemia

- Q. What is done for nutrition ?
  - A diet rich in proteins and carbs is given to combat malnutrition
  - Fat-soluble vitamins
  - Avoid fat to reduce steatorrhea
- Q. Enlist the pathogenic factors for FCPD.
  - Malnutrition
  - Protein deficiency
  - Cassava toxicity
  - Oxidative stress
  - Genetic and familial causes
- Q. Which are the cyanogenic glycosides present in cassava?
  - Linamarin
  - Lotaustralin
- Q. What are the investigations done to diagnose FCPD?
  - Tests to detect pancreatic function-
  - Test to detect pancreatic morphology - Xray, USG, EUS, ERCP, etc
- Q. Which are the tests to detect pancreatic function?
  - Fecal elastase
  - Fecal chymotrypsin
  - Fecal immunoreactive lipase
- Q. Enlist the complications associated with FCPD.
  - Pancreatic cancer- 100 times increased risk
  - Retinopathy and other microvascular complications
  - Pancreatic osteodystrophy malnutrition + malabsorption + diabetes = severe osteoporosis
  - Pancreatic exocrine deficiency
- Q. Enlist the treatment options for FCPD.
  - Diabetes management
  - Exocrine pancreatic enzyme replacement
  - Fat-soluble vitamin replacement- intramuscularly
  - Pain management
  - Endotherapy- ESWL + ERCP

    - Early cancer detection
    - Surgical therapy- mainly for the pain

- Q. Is malnutrition a cause or effect of FCPD?

    - Recent studies suggest malnutrition is an effect rather than the cause of FCPD

- Q. Enlist the various theories for FCPD over time?

    - Cassava theory Geerverghese and McMillin
    - Increase oxidative stress theory
    - Genetic theory recent theory

- Q. Which genetic mutation has been associated with FCPD ?

    - SPINK1
    - PRSS1 and PRSS2
    - Chymotrypsinogen C

- Q. Diabetes onset is at what age?

    - Generally aged 20-30 years
    - About 1-2 decades after the first episode of abdominal pain

- Q. Is insulin secretory defect established in FCPD?

    - Yes

- Q. Is the exocrine and endocrine deficiency linked?

    - It seems from some of the studies done by Yajnik et al

- Q. What is the newer paradigm in the etiology of diabetes in FCPD?

    - New interest in FCPD is directed to insulin resistance as a cause of diabetes in FCPD

- Q. What is the link between insulin resistance and chronic pancreatitis?

    - Some studies have shown that patients with pancreatic diabetes have hepatic insulin resistance due to the internalization of hepatic insulin receptors and GLUT2
    - The role of the pancreatic polypeptide has also been proposed

- Q. What is the role of a pancreatic polypeptide?

    - Studies have shown that pancreatic polypeptide regulates the expression of the IR gene in the liver
    - Thus impairment of PP will impair glucose homeostasis via IR gene expression in the liver

- Q. Do patients with FCPD have insulin resistance similar to Type 2 diabetes patients?

    - Yes
    - This is according to a study by Mohan et al
    - So FCPD patients have insulin resistance similar to type 2 diabetics!

- Q. Is the BMI in these patients showing something else?

    - Singla et al. showed that these patients have higher body fat percentage despite low BMI
    - This could contribute to insulin resistance

- Q. What is the vicious cycle of glucagon and insulin?

    - As far as 35 years ago, it was proposed that diabetes is not just an insulin problem but also a problem with glucagon
    - Insulin resistance increases insulin production and secretion → higher intra-islet insulin concentration → increases glucagon production → further increases insulin secretion → vicious circle

- Q. Is glucagon indeed depleted in patients with FCPD?

    - This theory is questioned now
    - Some studies by Mohan and Yajnik have shown that FCPD may have preserved glucagon response and selective damage to beta cells

- Q. What is the role of incretin hormones in the pathogenesis of diabetes in chronic pancreatitis

    - Knop et al. suggested that CP without diabetes had an intact incretin response compared to CP with diabetes
    - This may be the missing link in FCPD
    - Also, he showed that pancreatic enzyme replacement might augment incretin response- a theory that could have an impact on the management of FCPD

- Q. What is the role of body composition causing diabetes in FCPD?

    - There is a theory that the lack of fat tissue may be due to the lipodystrophy-like effect, which can lead to insulin resistance in FCPD patients
    - Deficiency fat stores increase hepatic triglyceride stores → increase circulating fatty acids → improve insulin resistance

ÞÞÞ

Real-life-cases

- A 30-year-old male presented with a history of unintentional weight loss
- His weight reduced from 100 kg to 70 kg over 3 months
- During this process, the patient was found to have hyperglycemia
- The patient was started on insulin, and some weight was regained but over a few weeks he started developing hypoglycemia
- Insulin was stopped and the patient was started on Oral antidiabetics by his physician

- At the age of 25, he had recurrent episodes of abdominal pain which were never investigated
- When he came to us he had an HbA1c of 10%
- Looking at the unusual history, we decided to perform a CT scan of the abdomen
- True to what we suspected, we found the pancreas studded with calcification
- There was no evidence of malignancy - however, the risk and screening for the same have been explained to the patient
- The patient was restarted on insulin and pancreatic enzyme supplementation along with nutritional replenishment
- Currently, he has regained some weight and maintains good glycemic control

Things to learn from the case:

- Sometimes a diagnosis of FCPD can be made retrospectively!
- In patients with acute symptomatic hyperglycemia- if the [[Glucose Toxicity (Glucotoxicity)]] breaks- the patient can start developing hypoglycemia. The risk of hypoglycemia is higher in patients with FCPD
- Abdominal pain can disappear over some time. At later age, the patient may present with just exocrine and endocrine insufficiency
- This patient is from Rajasthan. FCPD is not restricted to some regions of the country and can be considered a pan-Indian issue

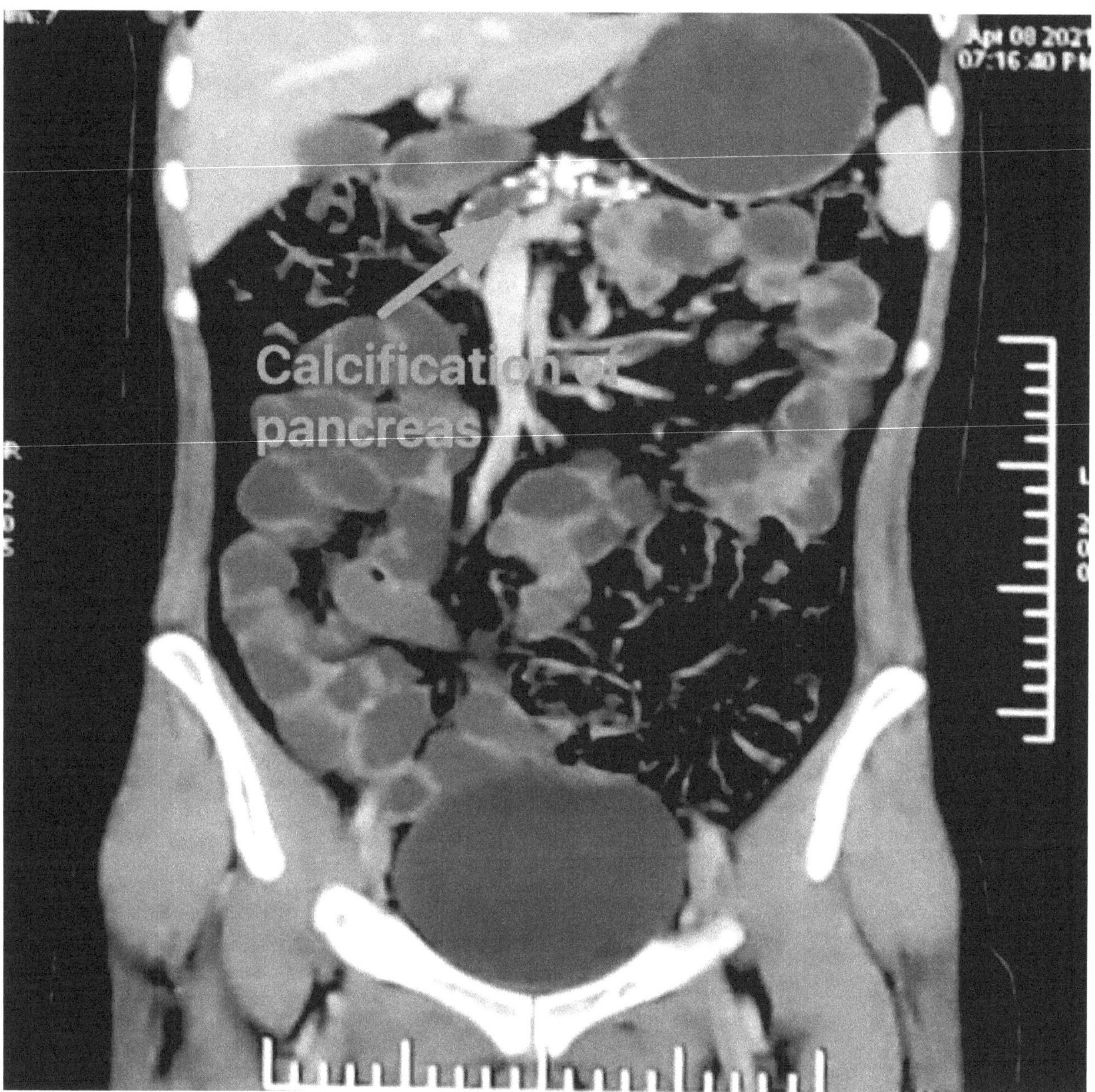

Figure 10.1: A Real-life case of FCPD

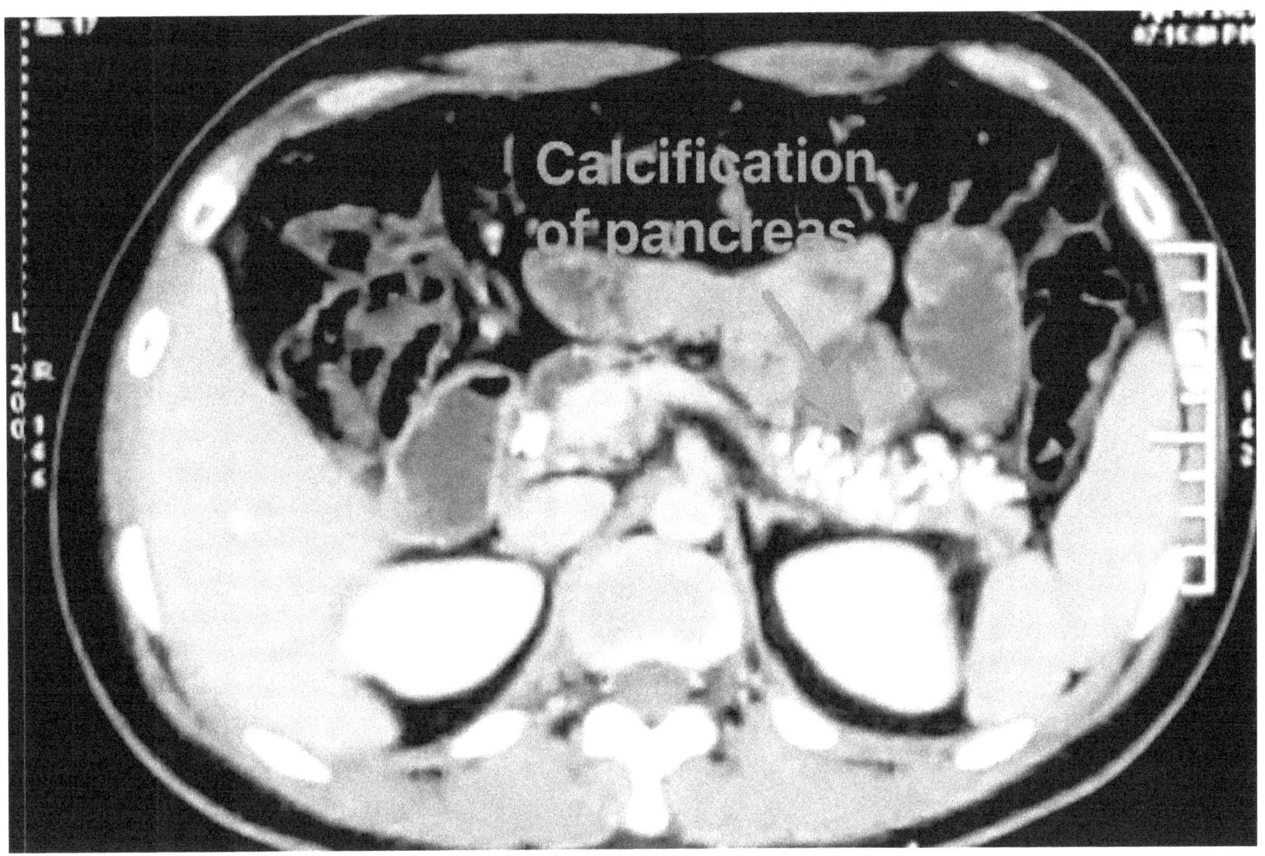

Figure 10.2: A Real-life case of FCPD

ELEVEN

Latent autoimmune diabetes of Adulthood (LADA)

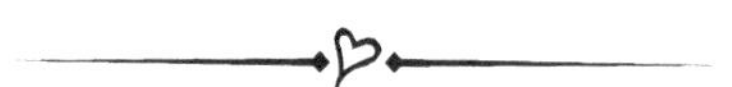

- Q. What are the diagnostic criteria for Latent autoimmune diabetes of Adulthood (LADA) ?

    - Age > 30 years
    - At least 1 insulin cell autoantibodies positive
    - Period of 6 months on insulin independence

- Q. What are the expanded clinical criteria for Latent autoimmune diabetes of Adulthood (LADA) ?

    - Age at onset > 30 years
    - A family or personal history of autoimmunity
    - A reduced frequency of metabolic syndrome compared with people with full-on type 2 diabetes: lower HOMA, lower body mass index, lower blood pressure, normal HDL compared with people with type 2 diabetes
    - No disease-specific difference in cardiovascular outcomes between these patients and those with type 2 diabetes
    - C-peptide levels fall more slowly than in traditional type 1 diabetes
    - Positivity for anti-GAD antibodies is the most sensitive marker, but other autoantibodies can be found as well, just less frequently
    - Noninsulin-requiring at the onset

- Q. Which is the preferred marker to diagnose LADA?

    - Anti GAD65

- Q. What are the subtypes of LADA?

    - LADA1 is a lesser C peptide, more ketosis-prone, and higher GAD antibody
    - LADA2- greater C peptide, less ketosis-prone, lesser GAD antibody positivity

- Q. What is LADY?

    - Latent autoimmune diabetes in Young
    - Similar to LADA but age is <30 years

- Q. What is the importance of a positive GAD antibody in any diabetic individual?
  - Positive GAD antibody in any diabetic predicts the requirement for early insulin requirement
- Q. Which is the latest antibody for Type 1 Diabetes or Latent autoimmune diabetes of Adulthood (LADA)?
  - Tetraspanin 7
- Q. Are there any benefits of early insulin initiation?
  - Yes
  - Early insulin initiation would help give rest to beta-cells and give overall good control
- Q. Which heat shock protein has been found to reduce beta-cell destruction?
  - Diapep 277- a heat shock protein 60 derivative has been found to reduce the incidence of beta-cell destruction in both type 1 diabetes and LADA
- Q. What vaccine has been found to retard beta-cell damage?
  - Anti GAD65 vaccine DIAMYD
- Q. How do these vaccines work?
  - They cause a shift from pro-inflammatory Th1 cells to anti-inflammatory Th2 cells
  - This shift suppresses the cytokine produced by Th1
  - This is a form of "acquired immune tolerance"
- Q. What is the core difference between adult type 1 diabetes and LADA?
  - The core difference is the speed of the beta-cell destruction leading to the dependency on insulin
  - Adult-onset Type 1 Diabetes has more rapid beta-cell destruction unlike LADA
  - This is differentiated by the criteria which say 6 or more months of insulin independence after onset which is required for LADA
    - If insulin requirement is before 6 months - it is adult type 1
    - otherwise, it is LADA
- Q. Which OAD must be avoided for use in LADA?
  - Avoid sulphonylurea
- Q. Can other OAD be used in LADA?
  - Yes
  - There are small studies for the benefit of all other OADs including SGLT2i in LADA patients
- Q. Should all patients with Type 2 Diabetes mellitus be screened for LADA?

- Yes
- According to the recent guidelines on the topic

- Q. Give the algorithm for diagnosis and management of Latent autoimmune diabetes of Adulthood (LADA)

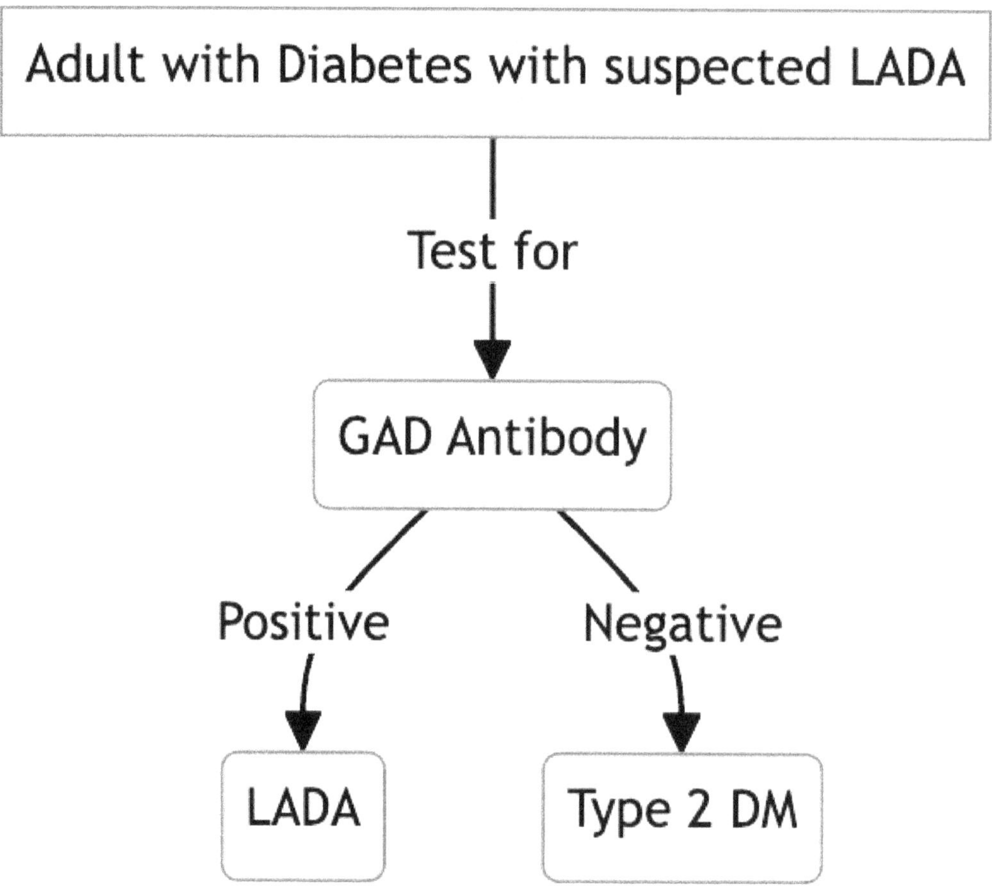

Figure 11.1 Algorithm for LADA. Step 1

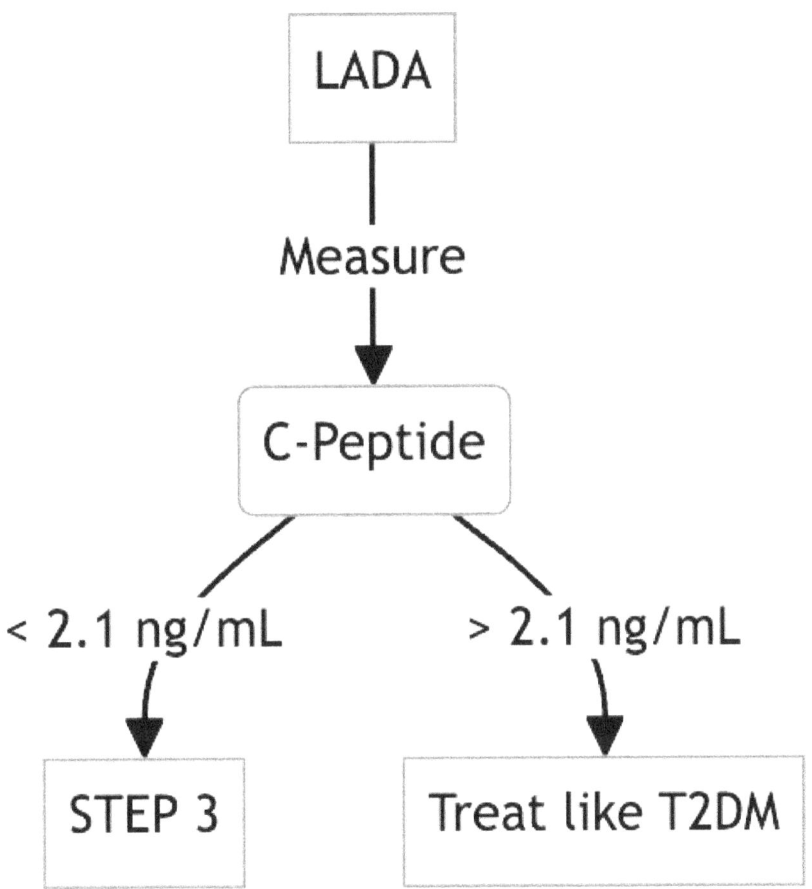

Figure 11.2 Algorithm for LADA step 2

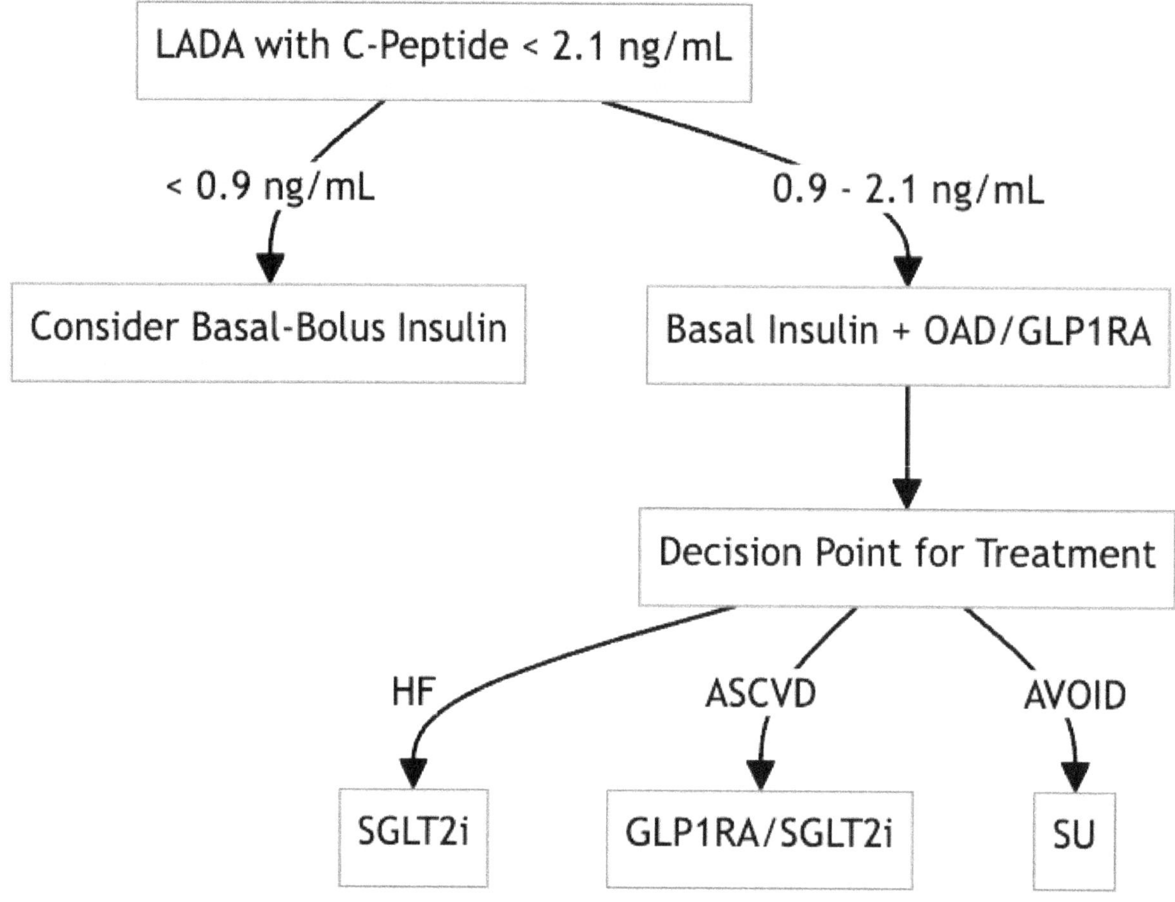

Figure 11.3 Algorithm for LADA Step 3OAD: Oral antidiabetic, HF: Heart failure, ASCVD: Atherosclerotic cardiovascular disease

- Q. What is the C-peptide-based approach to the management of a patient with LADA?
  - C-peptide
    - <0.9 ng/ml (0.3 nmol/l) - The patient should be on basal-bolus insulin
    - 0.9-2.1 ng/ml (0.3-0.7 nmol/l) - The patient should be on basal insulin plus OAD
    - More than 2.1 ng/ml (>0.7 nmol/l) - treat with OAD and as per the ADA guidelines for type 2 diabetes
- Q. What should be the glucose levels while performing the C-peptide assay?
  - 80-180 mg/dl
- Q. Apart from the insulin requirement and OAD, which other factors must be kept in mind when a patient has LADA instead of Type 2 Diabetes mellitus?
  - Increased risk of other autoimmune diseases - including hypothyroidism

- Q. What were the conclusions from the Botnia study group published in 2010?
  - The study was done to look at the impact of GAD antibodies in the future risk of diabetes in non-diabetic individuals
  - The study found the following:
    - GADA positivity is a strong predictor of diabetes, regardless of family history.
    - People with high GADA concentrations are at an increased risk of developing diabetes.
    - GADA positivity tends to occur in families with type 1 diabetes or latent autoimmune diabetes in adults.
    - Low or medium levels of GADA do not impact the incidence of diabetes in individuals without a family history of diabetes.
    - Elevated GADA concentrations indicate an increased risk of diabetes in both relatives and control subjects.
    - The risk of diabetes is influenced by age, sex, BMI, GADAs, and family history of type 1 or type 2 diabetes.
    - GADA positivity significantly raises the risk of diabetes, in addition to traditional risk factors for type 2 diabetes
- Q. What level of GAD65 antibody was considered as positive in this study ?
  - Levels of about 32 IU/l were considered positive
- Q. Should patients with LADA be given SU? Does it impact long-term beta-cell reserve?
  - A study published in JCEM concluded that it is better to give insulin early and not Sulphonylurea in patients with LADA
  - A study conducted by Taro Maruyama et al. focused on comparing the effectiveness of insulin therapy versus sulfonylurea (SU) treatment in preserving or reversing beta-cell function in patients with slowly progressive insulin-dependent diabetes or LADA.
  - The study was a randomized clinical trial that included 60 patients with a 5-year duration or shorter of diabetes.
  - The primary endpoint of the study was an insulin-dependent state defined by low levels of serum C-peptide values.
  - The results showed that the progression rate to an insulin dependent state was lower in the insulin group compared to the SU group, indicating that insulin therapy may be more effective in preserving beta-cell function in LADA patients.

PPP

References:

1. Buzzetti R, Tuomi T, Mauricio D, Pietropaolo M, Zhou Z, Pozzilli P, Leslie RD. Management of Latent Autoimmune Diabetes in Adults: A Consensus Statement From an International Expert Panel. Diabetes. 2020 Oct;69(10):2037-2047. doi: 10.2337/dbi20-0017. Epub 2020 Aug 26. PMID: 32847960; PMCID: PMC7809717.
2. Maruyama T, Tanaka S, Shimada A, Funae O, Kasuga A, Kanatsuka A, Takei I, Yamada S, Harii N, Shimura H, Kobayashi T. Insulin intervention in slowly progressive insulin-dependent (type 1) diabetes mellitus. The Journal of Clinical Endocrinology & Metabolism. 2008 Jun 1;93(6):2115-21.

TWELVE

MECHANISM OF BETA-CELL DYSFUNCTION IN TYPE 2 DIABETES MELLITUS

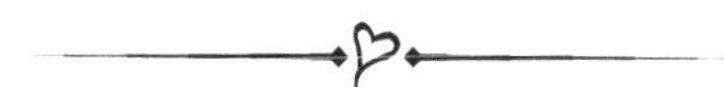

- Q. How many islets of Langerhans do we have and how many Beta-cells in each of them?
    - We have 1 million islets of langerhans
    - Each islet has 1000 Beta-cells
- Q. What percentage of Beta-cells function is lost at the time of diagnosis of Type 2 Diabetes mellitus and what percentage is lost every year?
    - 50% is lost at the time of diagnosis
    - 4-5% reduction every year
- Q. What does insulin output depend upon?
    - It depends upon
        1. beta-cell mass
        2. beta-cell function
- Q. What is the current debate on the role of Beta-cells in Type 2 diabetes?
    - The current debate is whether is there a reduction in beta-cell mass that leads to type 2 diabetes or it is a reduction in beta-cell function that leads to diabetes
- Q. Why is this debate important?
    - This is important because if there is only loss of function and not mass to potential of remission from disease is high
    - However, if there is a loss of mass and less issue with function- the potential of remission over the long term is questionable

- Q. What are Swisa's models for Beta-cell failure in Type 2 Diabetes mellitus?

    - Reduced beta-cell number
    - Beta-cell dysfunction due to (Also called beta-cell exhaustion)
    - Endoplasmic reticulum stress
    - Oxidative stress
    - Compromised identity of Beta-cells
    - Dedifferentiation/transdifferentiation of beta-cells

- Q. First model - What leads to reduction of reduced beta-cell mass?

    - People may have low beta-cells to begin with (Fetal programming)
    - Beta-cells may undergo apoptosis
    - Aging leads to a decline in beta-cell mass

- Q. Second model - What leads to reduced beta-cell function ?

    - Endoplasmic reticulum stress
    - Endoplasmic reticulum stress is an important cause of beta-cell loss in both type 1 and Type 2 Diabetes mellitus
    - Oxidative stress

  - This is where the phenomenon of Glucose Toxicity (Glucotoxicity) comes into the picture
  - This is the recoverable part of Beta-cell dysfunction
  - There might be temporary stunning of beta-cells due to Hyperglycemia

- Q. Of the above two models - which is more important?

  - Model 2 (reduced beta-cell function) is more important
  - This is because the reduction of beta-cell mass can be compensated by an increase in beta-cell function
  - A patient can have diabetes even with normal beta-cell mass
  - On the contrary- an increase of beta-cell mass may not always compensate for reduced beta-cell function
  - This is a very important thing to understand

- Q. According to a study, which drugs lead to how much monotherapy failure?

  - At 5 years

    - Glyburide- 34%
    - Metformin- 21%
    - Rosiglitazone- 15%

- Q. Enlist the various tests that are useful for the Assessment of beta-cell function (beta-cell function) in clinical practice.

    - Proinsulin: Insulin ratio
    - HOMA-Beta
    - Mixed meal stimulation test

    - OGTT

- Q. What are the usual C-peptides in Fasting and post-meal states in euglycemic individual?

  - Fasting - 0.9-1.8 ng/ml
  - Post-meal- 3-9 ng/ml

- Q. What is the best cut of blood C-peptide levels to determine insulin use in a post-prandial sample?

  - 2 hours post meal- C-peptide <6 ng/dl (<2.02 nmol/l) is a strong predictor of insulin requirement

- Q. What is the interpretation of Random C-peptide value?

  - The RBS >140 mg/dl for interpretation
  - Random c-peptide

    - <0.6 ng/ml ==> Absolute insulin deficiency
    - <1.8 ng/ml ==> Likely Type 1
    - 0.6-6.0 ng/ml ==> Requires mixed meal stimulation test
    - More than 6.0 ng/ml==> Rules out Type 1

  - Convert nmol/l to ng/dl by multiplying by 3

THIRTEEN

SECRETION OF INSULIN AND REGULATION OF INSULIN SECRETION

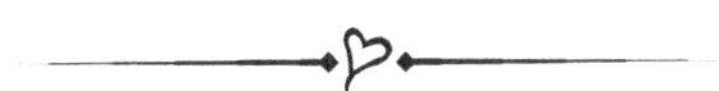

- Q. What are the different types of cells present in the endocrine pancreas?

Cells	Hormone released
Alpha cells	Glcuagon
Beta cells	Insulin
Delta cells	somatostatin
Gamma cells	pancreatic polypeptide
Episolon cells	ghrelin

Table 13.1: Types of Cells found in the pancreas and hormones released by them

- Q. Of these cells, which cell is the most abundant?
    - Beta-cells
    - They compose 60% of the islet cells
- Q. What are the differences between smaller islets and larger islets of the pancreas?
    - Smaller islets have more proportion of Beta-cells
    - they are closer to blood vessels
    - the release more insulin
- Q. How do beta-cells regenerate in the pancreas following extreme Beta-cells loss?
        - Neogenesis from Ductal cells
        - Transdifferentiation between Alpha cell and delta cells
        - Replication of beta-cells
- Q. What are the forms in which insulin is released in the human body?
    - Basal insulin secretion
        - Transcription factors play a role in the release of basal insulin
        - They are
        - HNF 4alpha
        - HNF1 alpha
        - IPF1
        - HNF 1 beta
        - NeuroD1
    - Nutrient-mediated insulin release
        - See below
- Q. Explain the process of nutrient-mediated insulin released from the pancreatic beta-cells.

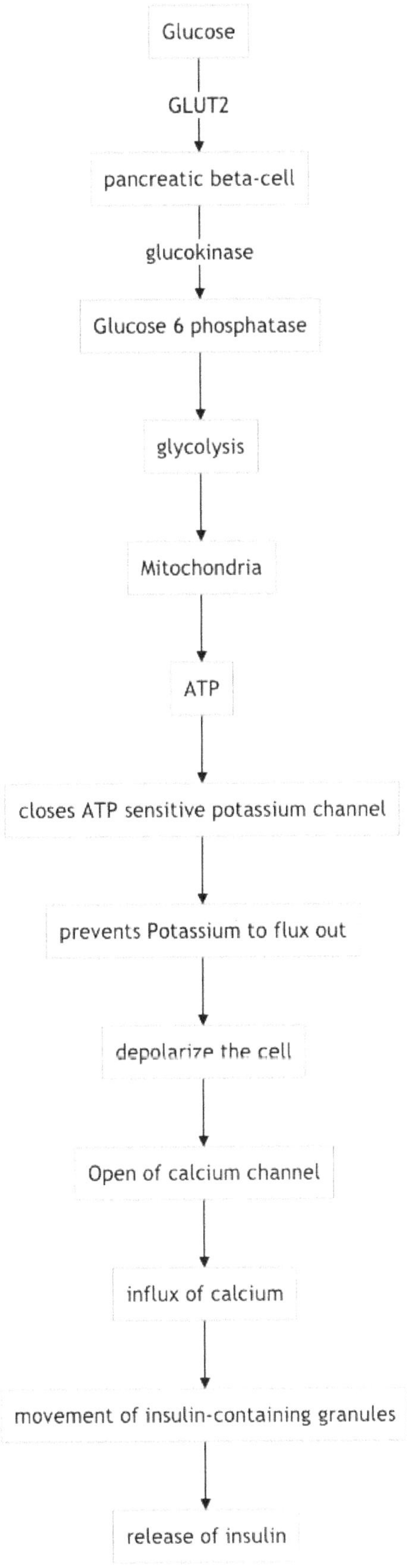

Figure 13.1: Nutrient-mediated release of insulin from beta-cells

- ***Clinical pearl***
    - *Closure/inhibition of K+ Channel releases insulin ....*
    - *If it remains open → neonatal diabetes*
    - *If it remains closed → hypoglycemia*

- Q. Can you tell us more about the biology of the ATP-sensitive potassium channels present in the beta-cells of the pancreas?
    - The SUR1-Kir6.2 pair constitutes the ATP-sensitive potassium channel
    - The SUR1 response to Sulphonylurea
    - The SUR1 is encoded by the ABCC8 gene
    - Closing of the ATP-sensitive potassium channel helps in the release of insulin
    - If the channel remains closed as in Loss of function mutation, it can produce hypoglycemia- as it occurs in Persistent hyperinsulinemic hypoglycemia of infancy
    - If the channel remains open (as it occurs in Gain-of-function mutation), it produces diabetes mellitus. This occurs in Neonatal diabetes mellitus

- Q. What is the role of cyclic-AMP second messenger in the release of insulin from beta-cells?
    - cAMP acts as an "amplifier" for insulin release
    - the action of cAMP is independent of the ATP-sensitive potassium channel, however, it is still a glucose-dependent system
    - The GLP-1 and GIP (The incretin) act via the cAMP pathway

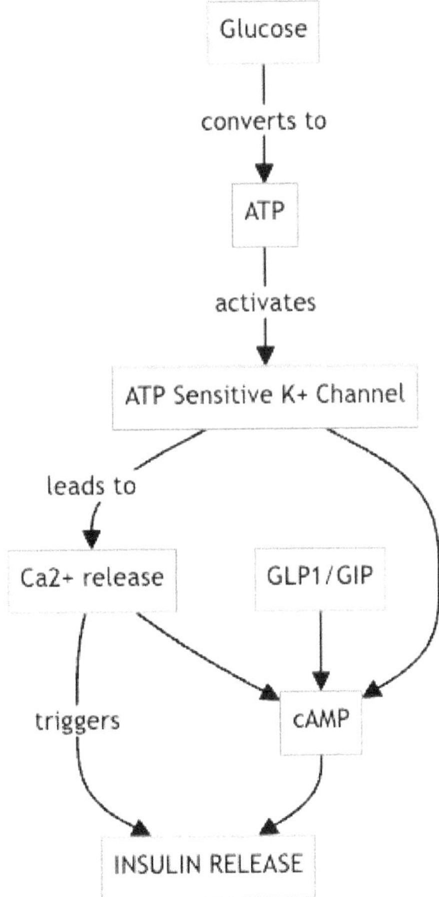

Figure 13.2: Figure shows how cAMP acts as an amplifier in the release of insulin

- Q. Are there any glucose sensors present in the pancreatic beta-cells that are independent of the glucose metabolism?
  - Yes. Other glucose sensors independent of glucose metabolism have been seen observed in rodent models. Two of them undergoing investigations currently are
    - Sweet taste receptors
    - Calcium sensory receptors
- Q. What is the importance of the sweet taste receptors?
  - Interestingly, sweet taste receptors are present in the pancreatic beta-cells of the human islets
  - Though their role in human islets is still under investigation, in rodent models they have been found to release insulin independent of the glucose metabolism.
  - Studies done in Wistar rats have shown that the "sweet taste" stimulates the release of insulin early on. This is also called the " Cephalic phase insulin release ".
  - As discussed above, their role in human beings is yet to be studied, but is is an interesting area of research.
- Q. What is the first-phase and second-phase insulin secretion?

  - Acute glycemia after a meal leads to an immediate burst release of preformed insulin → this is the first phase of insulin secretion
  - This is followed by slow and sustained release of insulin- 2nd phase insulin secretion which lasts for 1-2 hours

- Q. In what time frame is 1st phase of insulin released?

  - 1st phase insulin in response to glucose occurs within 3-5 min and subsides in 10 min

- Q. What is the periodicity of basal insulin secretion?

  - Insulin bursts are released every 11-14 min
  - Loss of pulsatility of basal insulin secretion is the first thing that is lost in the case of type 1 diabetes

- Q. What is the earliest change in insulin secretion seen in type 2 diabetes?

  - Loss of 1st phase insulin secretion

  - *Clinical pearl*

    - *Loss of pulsatility of basal insulin is 1st defect in type 1 diabetes*
    - *Loss of 1st phase of insulin secretion is the first defect in type 2 diabetes*

- Q. Which region of the brain is involved in the neural regulation of the beta-cell function?

  - The Hypothalamus

- Q. What is the impact of the autonomic nervous system on the beta-cell function?

  - The sympathetic system via alpha-2 receptor blocks the release of insulin and enhances glucagon release
  - The parasympathetic system vias the M3 muscarinic receptor enhances the release of insulin and suppresses glucagon release

BETA-CELL MASS

- Q. What is the beta-cell mass?

  - Beta-cell mass is the net amount of beta-cell
  - the net mass be reduced by some factors and increased by some factors

- Q. What factors reduce the beta-cell mass?

  - Beta-cell apoptosis
  - Dedifferentiation to alpha and other cells

- Q. What factors increase the beta-cell mass?
    - Neogenesis from Ductal cells
    - Transdifferentiation between Alpha cell and delta cells
    - Replication of beta-cells
- Q. What is the average life span of beta-cells?
    - 25 years
- Q. What are "virgin" beta-cells?
    - In the peripheral of the islet, there is a pool of immature or virgin beta-cell that can transdifferentiate into either alpha or beta-cells depending on the microenvironment
    - this can be a potential lifelong reservoir of beta-cells

ÞÞÞ

BETA-CELLS INSULIN CONTENT

- Q. How much of an insulin reservoir does the pancreas have at any given point of time ?
    - In normal healthy lean individuals, the pancreas has a reserved of 200-250 units of insulin at any given time which is enough to last for about 10 days
- Q. Where is the insulin stored within the beta-cells?
    - Insulin is stored within about 5000 secretory granules present in the beta-cells of the pancreas
- Q. Can you tell us about the basic structure of an insulin granule?
    - The insulin granule has an electron-dense core that contains insulin packed in hexamers
    - On the outside, there is one calcium and two zinc ions which stabilize this core
- Q. What percentage of granule insulin is secreted in response to glucose?
    - Only a small fracture of granule insulin (<1%) is secreted in response to glucose stimulation
- Q. What is the half-life of an insulin granule?
    - It is just about 5 days
- Q. What is the difference between younger and older granules?
    - Younger granules are more mobile than older granules

ÞÞÞ

MEASURES OF INSULIN SECRETION AND BETA-CELL MASS

- Q. What are the various methods for measuring insulin secretion?
    - OGTT and IVGTT
    - Measuring insulin levels
    - Arginine-induced glucose secretion
- Q. Which of these tests correlate best with beta-cell mass?
    - Insulin response to glucose and arginine correlate best with beta-cell mass
- Q. Which nuclear imaging technique is being developed to assess beta-cell mass?
    - PET Scan
- Q. How much beta cell mass is lost before fasting blood glucose starts to rise?
    - 60-70% of the beta-cell mass is lost
- Q. Is insulin measurement a good test for the assessment of beta-cell mass?
    - No
    - Because insulin resistance greatly determines insulin level, fasting insulin level is not a great test for beta-cell mass
- Q. What is AIRgluc?
    - It is an acute insulin response to glucose
    - It is a good test for the assessment of beta-cell mass
    - IV glucose is given and the amount of rising insulin in 10 min is measured
    - This measures the first phase insulin response
    - People at risk of type 2 / type 1 diabetes have less insulin secretion in 1st 10 min (loss of 1st phase insulin response) compared to normal people
- Q. What is a hallmark in response to various stimuli in type 2 diabetes?
    - In type 2 diabetes 1st phase insulin response to glucose is lost but the response to arginine or isoproterenol is maintained
    - This is the hallmark of type 2 diabetes

ꟼꟼꟼ

INSULIN SECRETION VERUS PLASMA INSULIN

- Q. What is insulin predominantly secreted?
  - Insulin is predominantly released into the portal circulation
- Q. What is C-peptide?
  - The pancreatic proinsulin is broken down into insulin and C-peptide
  - the C-peptide is released in equimolar concentration as insulin
- Q. Why is C-peptide a better measure of insulin secretion?
  - This is because of the following reasons:
    - a) The amount of C-peptide that is released is equal to the amount of insulin release
    - b) C-peptide is NOT extracted by the liver whereas the majority of endogenous insulin is extracted by the liver (remember insulin is released into the portal circulation)
    - c) C-peptide clearance accounts via the kidney - but this is constant. That means at any given point in time, the amount cleared by the kidney is constant to the amount that is being produced
    - d) Exogenous insulin does not impact the measure of c-peptide hence c-peptide is a measure of endogenous insulin production
- Q. Can you calculate the exact amount of insulin being secreted by measuring the C-peptide levels?
  - Yes.
  - Using a mathematical process can Deconvolution you can measure an approximate amount of insulin that is secreted by measuring the C-peptide
- Q. What is Deconvolution?
  - This is an algorithm-based process in which the recorded data can be reversed and engineered to find the original signal
  - This is based on the theory that the recorded data or signal is the original signal which is then filtered
  - So basically by measuring the C-peptide you can trace it back to its root and find the amount of insulin that is secreted
- Q. Does the C-peptide measured in the urine correlate with insulin secretion?
  - Yes
  - Urine c-peptide to creatinine ratio (UCPCR) gives a good estimate of beta-cell reserve in patients with Type 1 Diabetes
  - It is typically measured 2 hours after a meal
  - The sample is collected using boric acid as a preservative
  - UCPCR value <0.2 nmol/mmol is strongly suggestive of absolute insulin deficiency as seen in long-standing Type 1 Diabetes

CHARACTERISTICS OF INSULIN SECRETION IN VIVO

- Q. Under normal physiological conditions which is more stable insulin sensitivity or insulin secretion?
    - Insulin sensitivity is relatively stable in normal physiological conditions. The insulin sensitivity only varies by 30 to 80% throughout the 24 hour period. Pharmacologically, we can improve insulin sensitivity only by as much as 2 times the baseline.
    - Insulin secretion on the other hand can vary throughout the day and can vary based on the meal which is taken. You can improve insulin secretion by manyfold in the same individual.
- Q. As a gross figure how much insulin is required to dispose of 75 g of glucose in a lean individual vis-a-vis an obese individual?
    - According to William's textbook of endocrinology, 0.5 units of insulin is required to dispose of 75 g of glucose in an insulin-sensitive lean individual.
    - In an obese insulin-resistant individual this figure is as high as 45 units.
- Q. What is an ' insulinogenic index ' ?
    - The insulinogenic index is the simplest marker of first phase insulin secretion
    - It is calculated using an OGTT
    - It is the ratio of the change of insulin secretion in 30 minutes from baseline to post glucose load divided by the change in glucose value during this period
        - IGI = δinsulin (0-30 min)/δglucose (0-30 min)
            - (Insulin is measured in microunits per milliliter, whereas glucose is measured in milligrams per decilitre)

ᑭᑭᑭ

MODES OF BETA-CELL RESPONSE

- Q. Give an outline of insulin secretion in the human body.

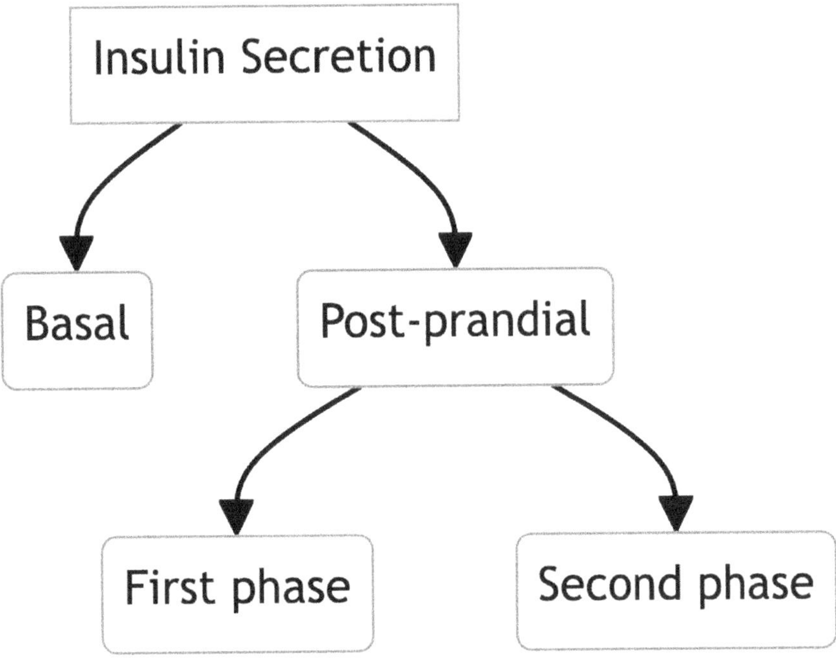

Figure 13.3 Outline for insulin secretion in the human body

- Q. What are the three main modes of Beta-cell response (insulin secretory response) ?
  - First-phase insulin secretion
  - Beta-cell glucose sensitivity
  - Potentiation of insulin secretion
- Q. What is the First phase of insulin secretion?
  - Insulin release occurs in two ways
    - Basal- continuous insulin that is released from the beta-cell irrespective of the food or glucose intake
    - Post-meal insulin release
  - In the post-meal insulin release- there is an acute response to glucose upsurge that occurs within 2 minutes of glucose excursion which is called the first-phase insulin secretion
  - This is a burst of insulin secretion that occurs from preformed and mature insulin secretory granules
  - This is a form of pre-emptive method of preventing a glucose surge. This first phase suppresses hepatic glucose production and enhances the peripheral glucose utilization
  - The First phase of insulin secretion can be assessed by
    - Hyperglycemic clamp
    - Intravenous glucose tolerance test IVGTT
- Q. What is the second phase of insulin secretion?

- It is the slow and sustained release of insulin post the glucose load
- This is derived mainly from the reserve pool of insulin granules

- ***Pearl***
  - *First phase insulin- from readily releasable pool (RRP)*
  - *Second phase insulin- from the reserve pool*

- Q. In terms of the new theory, how do we subdivide the RRP into three parts?
  - "Old Face"- these are docked granules ready to be released. They are already docked and released as soon as the signal arrives.
  - "The restless newcomer"- they are newly recruited on stimulation and are fuse almost immediately to the plasma membrane
  - "The resting newcomer"- they are recruited on stimulation but are first docked (rested) and then they fuse to the plasma membrane and released
  - All three contribute the the first phase of insulin secretion

- Q. What is Beta-cell glucose sensitivity?
  - As discussed earlier, the Beta-cells sense the glucose excursion and release insulin in response to the same
  - In that regard, beta-cell is both a sensor of glucose and a producer of insulin
  - Beta-cell glucose sensitivity is the measure of the ability of the beta-cell to sense the glucose
  - There is a school of thought that the Beta-cell glucose sensitivity is one of the early defects that occur in patients with Type 2 Diabetes
  - ie if the glucose cannot be sensed properly, how will insulin be released in response to the same
  - Naturally, the First phase of insulin secretion is affected by the same.

- Q. What is the potentiation of insulin secretion?
  - In a normal beta-cell insulin secretion is potentiated in accordance to the glucose levels
  - other factors like incretins, fructose, Sulphonylurea etc may also help in the potentiation

- Q. Apart from glucose what are the other nutrient factors that impact insulin release?
  - Some amino acids like Arginine and Free Fatty acid also potentiate insulin release apart from the glucose

- Q. Is basal insulin secreted in a pulsatile manner?
  - Yes
  - Basal insulin is secreted in short bursts of 5-14 minutes
  - Over 24 hours there are also 80-180 minute ultradian cycles

- Q. What happens to the pulsatile secretion in a hyperglycemic state?
  - The pulsatile secretion is disrupted in a hyperglycemic state

- Q. What is the importance of Prolinsulin to insulin ratio?

  - The higher proinsulin to insulin or proinsulin to c-peptide ratio is a marker of beta-cell dysfunction and risk of diabetes mellitus

ঌঌঌ

INSULIN SECRETORY RESPONSE TO INTRAVENOUS GLUCOSE

- Q. What is the Hyperglycemic clamp?
  - This is a study done to assess the first-phase and second-phase insulin response
  - Here the person is given an acute burst of glucose
  - Initially, there is a sharp increase in glucose secretion. This is the first phase of insulin secretion
  - Then there is a small dip in insulin release
  - This is followed by a slow and sustained release of insulin again- which is the second phase of insulin secretion
- Q. What is the typical magnitude of First-phase insulin secretion?
  - In a normal individual for a glucose upsurge of >126 mg/dl , the first phase insulin secretion (also called Acute insulin response) is typically 4 nmol/m2 of body surface area.
  - This is approximately 1 unit in a 70 kg man.
  - This is about 10% of the total insulin release in the second phase
- Q. Is it true the loss of first-phase insulin secretion is the earliest marker of Beta-cell dysfunction?
  - Yes.
  - That is correct

ঌঌঌ

INTRAVENOUS GLUCOSE TOLERANCE TEST IVGTT

- Q. What is IVGTT?
  - This is another method for assessment of First phase insulin secretion
  - Here the glucose is infused IV and the insulin and c-peptide are measured at regular intervals
  - Here the First phase insulin secretion is similar to Hyperglycemic clamp but the subsequent response (second phase) is different because of the different methodology
- Q. What is a Graded glucose infusion test?
  - This is a test for the dose-response relationship between insulin secretion and glucose infusion
  - ProSciento literature states the procedure as follows:

    - "After an overnight fast a basal (control) period is followed by sequential incremental intravenous infusions of glucose calculated to raise the blood glucose concentration from fasting levels to the hyperglycemic range (approximately 300mg/dL,17 mmol/L).
    - A graded infusion of 20% glucose is administered at 2, 4, 6, 8, and 12 mg/kg/min each for 30 minutes. Blood samples are drawn at 10, 20, and 30 minutes during each 30 minutes for measurement of glucose, insulin, and plasma C-peptide

  - This is used in research labs to generate pre-clinical data on the effectiveness of novel therapies in diabetes

- Q. In an individual with a good beta-cell reserve, does a mild chronic hyperglycemia, sustain insulin secretion?

  - Yes.
  - Graded glucose infusion tests have shown that in subjects with good beta-cell reserve, a chronic mild hyperglycemia can potentiate the insulin secretion and the body can maintain homeostasis.

REGULATION OF INSULIN SECRETION

- Q. Summarize the various factors that regular insulin secretion?

  - Nutrients that enhance insulin release

    - Glucose
    - Fatty acid
    - Amino acids

- Intra-islet hormones

  - Glucagon increases insulin
  - Somatostatin reduces insulin

- Neurotransmitter

  - Acetylcholine- increase insulin
  - Catecholamine

    - Via alpha2- reduce insulin
    - Via beta 2 increases insulin

- Gut hormones

  - Increase insulin

    - GLP1
    - GIP

        - VIP
        - Secretin
    - Reduce insulin
        - Ghrelin
- Adipokine
    - Increase insulin
        - adiponectin
    - Reduce insulin
        - Leptin
        - Resistin
- Other hormones
    - Increase insulin
        - Vitamin D
        - Estrogen
    - Reduce insulin
        - IGF1
        - Thyroid hormone
- Glucocorticoids have dual-action
    - directly reduce insulin but produce hyperglycemia which increases insulin
- Drugs
    - SU and GLL1 analog- increase insulin
    - Diazoxide reduce insulin
- Q. How do non-nutrient factors regulate insulin secretion?
    - Via cAMP eg: glucagon, GLP1
    - Via Phospholipase C CCK, Acetylcholine
- Q. What is the primary regulator of insulin secretion?
    - Glucose!

- Q. Apart from glucose, which other nutrients can potentially release insulin?
    - Amino acids
    - Fatty acids
- Q. Which amino acids enhance insulin secretion?
    - Glutamine + leucine
    - Arginine
- Q. What is the action of free fatty acid on insulin secretion?
    - Free fatty acid enhances Glucose stimulated insulin secretion
    - This probably compensates for the increased insulin resistance produced by free fatty acids in the initial stages
- Q. Which are two pools of insulin stored in secretory granules?
    - Readily releasable pool RRP – 1% - responsible for the 1st phase insulin release
    - Reserve pool - 99% - needs to undergo preparatory steps to be released
- Q. What is the effect of estradiol on insulin secretion?
    - Estradiol enhances insulin secretion
    - ER receptors are present on the pancreatic islets
- Q. What is the effect of melatonin on insulin secretion?
    - Newer studies have shown that melatonin inhibits insulin secretion
- Q. Which important gut hormone increases insulin secretion?
    - GLP1
- Q. Which other gut hormones increase insulin secretion?
    - CCK
    - VIP
    - Gastrin
    - GIP
    - Secretin
- Q. What is the effect of leptin on insulin secretion?
    - Leptin inhibits insulin secretion
- Q. What is the effect of IGF1 on insulin secretion?
    - IGF1 reduces insulin secretion

- Q What is the effect of thyroid hormone on insulin secretion?
    - It mildly reduces insulin secretion
- Q What is the effect of vitamin D on insulin secretion?
    - It enhances insulin secretion
- Q. What is the effect of glucocorticoid on insulin secretion?
    - Direct effect inhibits insulin secretion
    - The indirect effect increases insulin secretion by producing hyperglycemia and insulin resistance
- Q. What is the effect of catecholamines?
    - They inhibit insulin secretion by acting via alpha-receptors
    - However, beta 2 receptors - it enhances insulin secretion
- Q. What about somatostatin?
    - It inhibits insulin secretion
- Q. What about glucagon?
    - Increases insulin secretion
- Q. Summarize the impact of various drugs influencing insulin secretion.
    - Potassium channel blockers- SU and Meglitanitdes increase insulin secretion
    - Potassium channel openers- Diazoxide reduces insulin secretion
    - Calcium channel blockers- reduce insulin secretion, however, in vivo, they have little effect
    - GLP1 analog- enhances insulin secretion

FOURTEEN

Finerenone for Diabetic kidney disease

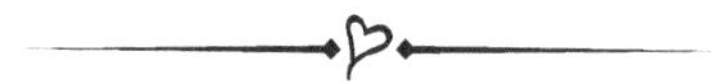

- Q. What is Finerenone ?
    - Finerenone, sold under the brand name Kerendia, is a medication used to reduce the risk of kidney function decline, kidney failure, cardiovascular death, non-fatal heart attacks, and hospitalization for heart failure in adults with chronic kidney disease associated with type 2 diabetes. Finerenone is a non-steroidal mineralocorticoid receptor antagonist(MRA)
- Q. How does Finerenone compare to other steroidal mineralocorticoid receptor antagonists MRA?
    - - It is a non-steroidal MRA
    - - It has high potency and is selective to mineralocorticoid receptor
    - - It has a short half-life of 2-3 hours
    - - Little effect on BP
    - - Less hyperkalemia
    - - No sexual side effects
    - - No CNS penetration
- Q. What is the dose of Finerenone?
    - 10 - 20 mg OD
- Q. What is the difference between FIDELIO-DKD and FIGARO-DKD?
    - FIDELIO-DKD looked at renal outcomes as the primary endpoint
    - FIGARO-DKD looked at CV outcomes as the primary endpoint
- Q. Which patients were included in these trials?
    - Albuminuria 30-300 with eGFR 25-90 - A2 + G1/G2/G3
    - Albuminuria >300 with eGFR - >60 - A3 + G1/G2
- Q. What was the duration of the follow-up of these patients?

    - It was 2-3 years

- Q. What was the main driver of the CV benefit in the Finerenone group?
    - Reduction of hospitalization due to heart failure

- Q. What were the renal end points studied?
    1. Kidney failure- defined as eGFR <15
    2. Sustained >40% reduction in eGFR from baseline
    3. Renal death

- Q. How much potassium increase is expected?
    - 0.2 meq/l

- Q. What is a FIDELITY study?
    - This was a pooled analysis of the two studies

- Q. What is the indication of Finerenone as per the AACE guideline?
    1. Type 2 diabetes
    2. eGFR- >25
    3. UACR >30
    4. On maximum dose of RAAS blocker

- Q. What should be the baseline potassium level before starting Finerenone?
    - <4.8 - can start
    - 4.8-5.0- caution
    - More than 5.0- Not recommended

- What should be the starting dose of Finerenone?
    - It is based on eGFR
    1. <25- not recommended
    2. 25-60- 10 mg OD
    3. More than 60- 20 mg OD

- Q. How should the dose be monitored based on potassium levels?
    - Potassium on follow-up
    1. <4.8- Can consider increasing to 20 mg if a patient is on 10 mg
    2. 4.8-5.5 - continue the same dose (10 or 20 mg)
    3. More than 5.5- stop treatment- restart if potassium <5.0

- Q. What are the 5, '5s' for Finerenone therapy?

    - initiate with eGFR >25
    - Initiate when potassium <5.0
    - With-hold when potassium >5.5
    - It reduces ESKD in 1 in 5 patients
    - It reduces heart failure risk in 1 in 5 patients

FIFTEEN

GLUCOSE TOXICITY (GLUCOTOXICITY)

- Q. Who was the first to give the concept of Glucose Toxicity (Glucotoxicity) ?
    - Rosetti and Defronzo
- Q. In the current sense what applies to Glucose Toxicity (Glucotoxicity) ?
    - In this chapter, it refers to excess glucose altering the mechanism of glucose itself
    - It is high glucose-producing Insulin resistance
- Q. What is the mass action of glucose?
    - This concept is the key to understanding Glucose Toxicity (Glucotoxicity)
    - What this means is, that in the presence of insulin, an increased level of glucose increases its uptake and utilization
    - This is dependent for insulin-dependent tissues and not on the tissues like brain
    - This is normal physiology in non-diabetic individuals
    - However, in diabetic individuals, the insulin production is reduced
    - Hence in such patients the glucose will increase and this hyperglycemia ideally would lead to increased glucose utilization overwhelming the patient
    - This does not happen because of a protective mechanism that the body has
    - In such a scenario, the body increases Insulin resistance leading to the normalization of glucose utilization in insulin-dependent tissues
    - So the insulin-dependent tissues are spared of the effect of the hyperglycemia, but what about the non-insulin-dependent tissues?
        - Now this WILL be affected
        - The effect is, however, restricted to tissues not protected by the blood-brain barrier - ie the brain again is spared
        - Which are these tissues? The big three- kidney, retina, and peripheral nerves!
- Q. What kind of Insulin resistance is seen in patients with Type 1 Diabetes?
    - Insulin resistance is mainly seen in the skeletal muscles peripheral insulin resistance

  - It is believed most of the insulin resistance in this case is attributable to Glucose Toxicity (Glucotoxicity)

- Q. Does Chronic hyperglycemia itself cause Diabetes mellitus?

  - Yes
  - This would be a consequence of Glucose Toxicity (Glucotoxicity)
  - Classical studies done in cats by Lukens and Dohan have shown that chronic hyperglycemia was responsible for causing permanent type 2 diabetes in these cats
  - Chronic hyperglycemia not only increases insulin resistance but also impairs beta-cell responsiveness to glucose
  - Studies have shown that hyperglycemia exposure for>68 hours leads to a significant reduction in insulin secretion
  - Interestingly in most of the animal studies, the use of phlorizin has been shown to restore the action- is there are role of SGLT2i in removing the Glucose Toxicity (Glucotoxicity)?

- Q. What are the potential mechanisms for Glucose Toxicity (Glucotoxicity) ?

    - Extra glucose -→ converted to Lipid -→ Lipid flux produces Insulin resistance
    - Increase Reactive oxygen species
    - Increase flux through hexosamine-linked glycation pathway

- Q. What is the importance of UDP-N-acetylglucosamine?

  - This is an intermediate which is an important nutrient sensor
  - All the glucose and other nutrients are converted to UDP-N-Acetylgluosamine via the hexosamine pathway

- Q. What is the link between Oxidative stress and Beta-cells damage?

  - Increased oxidative stress leads to Beta-cell dysfunction and damage
  - Remember oxidative stress also increases Insulin resistance

- Q. So in the case of Glucose Toxicity (Glucotoxicity) , is the response to other nutrients preserved?

  - This is the interesting part
  - In the case of Glucose Toxicity (Glucotoxicity), there is a loss of beta-cell response to glucose.
  - However, the beta-cell response to other nutrients that stimulate insulin release like Arginine is preserved and sometimes even exaggerated

- Q. What is the best example of Glucose Toxicity (Glucotoxicity) in Type 1 Diabetes?

  - The "honeymoon period" in Type 1 Diabetes

- Q. How common is the honeymoon period?

  - It is seen in almost 30% of patients with Type 1 Diabetes

- Q. What is an example of Glucose Toxicity (Glucotoxicity) in Type 2 Diabetes?

- The improvement in glycemic control and partial remission in Type 2 Diabetes because of Short-term intensive insulin therapy is an example of Glucose Toxicity (Glucotoxicity) in type 2 diabetes

"***Clinical pearl***

- *Glucose Toxicity (Glucotoxicity) leads to insulin resistance in both type 1 as well as type 2 diabetes which can be reversed with good glycemic control*

Connect With Us

You can connect with us in the following way

1. Email: dromlakhani@gmail.com
2. Website for Notes in Endocrinology: www.endocrinology.co.in
3. Website for our YouTube channel: https://www.youtube.com/@EndocrinologyIndia/videos
4. Twitter or X: https://twitter.com/omlakhani
5. Our other ongoing projects:

- a) EndoAl.co.in • The world's first and only large language model for Endocrinology
- b) Diabetology.co.in- Making diabetes care more algorithmic and hard-coded!
- c) Notes in Endocrinology Premium- Podcasts, AI, Workshops, CME and more

Purchasing volume 1:

About Best Of Notes In Endocrinology Volume 1

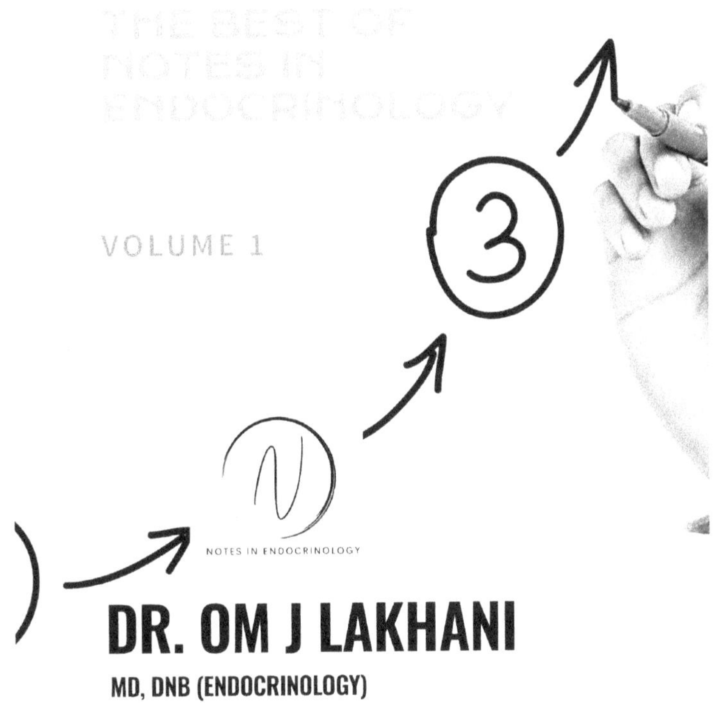

Enter Caption

The Number 1 Best Seller in the "Endocrinology" Category on Amazon!
Ordering the book (Print Edition):

1. NotionPress: https://notionpress.com/read/the-best-of-notes-in-endocrinology (Free Shipping)
2. Amazon: https://amzn.eu/d/fSVGHbB
3. Flipkart: https://www.flipkart.com/best-notes-endocrinology-volume-1/p/itm505589ccfcfed?pid=9798891860834&affid=editornoti

Chapters included in Volume 1:

1. Evidence-based Diets In Endocrinology, Diabetes & Metabolism
2. Aggressive Pituitary Tumor (Atypical Pituitary Tumor)
3. Pharmacological Management Of Obesity
4. Androgens And Cardiovascular Disease In Men
5. Refractory Hypothyroidism
6. Diagnosis Of Adrenal Insufficiency

7. Artificial Intelligence In Medicine
8. Imeglimin
9. Hypoglycemia In Adults Without Diabetes Mellitus

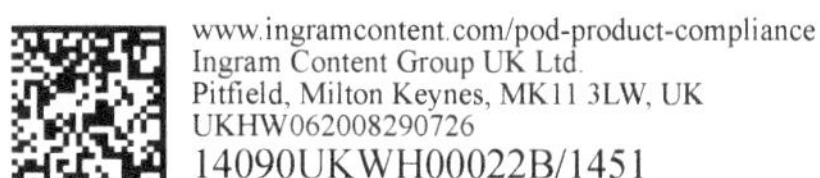
www.ingramcontent.com/pod-product-compliance
Ingram Content Group UK Ltd.
Pitfield, Milton Keynes, MK11 3LW, UK
UKHW062008290726
14090UKWH00022B/1451

9 798891 866430